COLOR ATLAS & SYNOPSIS OF CLINICAL OPHTHALMOLOGY
Wills Eye Institute

Retina

SECOND EDITION

Wolters Kluwer | Lippincott Williams & Wilkins
Health

Philadelphia · Baltimore · New York · London
Buenos Aires · Hong Kong · Sydney · Tokyo

Senior Executive Editor: Jonathan W. Pine, Jr.
Senior Product Managers: Emilie Moyer and Grace Caputo
Senior Manufacturing Coordinator: Benjamin Rivera
Marketing Manager: Lisa Lawrence
Creative Director: Doug Smock
Production Services: Aptara, Inc.

Printed in China

Library of Congress Cataloging-in-Publication Data
Retina / editors, Mitchell S. Fineman, Allen C. Ho. – 2nd ed.
    p. ; cm. – (Color atlas & synopsis of clinical
ophthalmology-Wills Eye Institute)
  Includes bibliographical references and index.
  ISBN 978-1-60913-336-8 (pbk. : alk. paper)
  I. Fineman, Mitchell S. II. Ho, Allen C. III. Wills Eye Hospital
(Philadelphia, Pa.)   IV. Series: Color atlas and synopsis of clinical
ophthalmology series.
  [DNLM: 1. Retinal Diseases–Atlases. WW 17]
  617.7′35–dc23

                          2011052818

Care has been taken to confirm the accuracy of the information presented and to describe generally accepted practices. However, the authors, editors, and publisher are not responsible for errors or omissions or for any consequences from application of the information in this book and make no warranty, expressed or implied, with respect to the currency, completeness, or accuracy of the contents of the publication. Application of the information in a particular situation remains the professional responsibility of the practitioner.

The authors, editors, and publisher have exerted every effort to ensure that drug selection and dosage set forth in this text are in accordance with current recommendations and practice at the time of publication. However, in view of ongoing research, changes in government regulations, and the constant flow of information relating to drug therapy and drug reactions, the reader is urged to check the package insert for each drug for any change in indications and dosage and for added warnings and precautions. This is particularly important when the recommended agent is a new or infrequently employed drug.

Some drugs and medical devices presented in the publication have Food and Drug Administration (FDA) clearance for limited use in restricted research settings. It is the responsibility of the health care provider to ascertain the FDA status of each drug or device planned for use in their clinical practice.

To purchase additional copies of this book, call our customer service department at (800) 638-3030 or fax orders to (301) 223-2320. International customers should call (301) 223-2300.

Visit Lippincott Williams & Wilkins on the Internet: at LWW.com. Lippincott Williams & Wilkins customer service representatives are available from 8:30 am to 6 pm, EST.

10 9 8 7 6 5 4 3 2 1

RRS1202

This edition is dedicated in memory of our colleague and mentor, J. Arch McNamara (1955–2010), whose clinical skills and passion for teaching will be missed by all who knew him, were inspired by him, and had the pleasure of his friendship.

Editors

Contributors

J. Luigi Borrillo, MD
Northern California Retina Vitreous Associates
  Medical Group
San Mateo, California

Richard S. Kaiser, MD
Associate Professor of Ophthalmology
Thomas Jefferson University
Attending Surgeon
Wills Eye Institute
Philadelphia, Pennsylvania

Nikolas J.S. London, MD
Fellow, Vitreoretinal Surgery
Wills Eye Institute
Philadelphia, Pennsylvania

Mithlesh C. Sharma, MD
Attending Vitreoretinal Surgeon
Kaiser Permanente Medical Group
Roseville, California

About the Series

The beauty of the atlas/synopsis concept is the powerful combination of illustrative photographs and a summary approach to the text. Ophthalmology is a very visual discipline that lends itself nicely to clinical photographs. Although the seven ophthalmic subspecialties in this series—Cornea, Retina, Glaucoma, Oculoplastics, Neuro-Ophthalmology, Pediatrics, and Uveitis—use varying levels of visual recognition, a relatively standard format for the text is used for all volumes. The goal of the series is to provide an up-to-date clinical overview of the major areas of ophthalmology for students, residents, and practitioners in all of the health care professions. The abundance of large, excellent quality photographs and concise, outline-form text will help achieve that objective.

Christopher J. Rapuano, MD
Series Editor

Preface

Vitreoretinal disease is a privileged visual discipline. There are significant barriers to its study beyond the constricted pupil. Ophthalmology trainees first acquire the observational skills and facility with diagnostic instrumentation such as the slit lamp biomicroscope and the indirect ophthalmoscope to begin to explore diseases that affect the posterior segment of the eye. It takes clinical experience to discern normal variation from significant pathology. Unfortunately, most nonophthalmic physicians are limited to facility with the direct ophthalmoscope that only affords a keyhole view of the back of the eye. We are privileged to be lifelong students, practitioners, clinical researchers and teachers of this aspect of the eye here at Wills Eye Hospital.

When we were asked to create a concise color atlas and synopsis of vitreoretinal disease we knew our challenges would be to be concise and to be selective since there is great richness of clinical detail, both visually and with words. Our aim was to balance the breadth of the subject material with enough focused detail to provide the framework of our thinking regarding important clinical signs, associated clinical signs, differential diagnosis, diagnostic evaluation, and prognosis and management of hundreds of vitreoretinal conditions. We want this to be a "go to" field manual but realize that it cannot be an encyclopedic reference.

The images of this color atlas and synopsis include over 300 color images and over 100 black and white images, typically fluorescein angiographic images. Each was digitized from an original photographic slide as a high resolution RGB image, at least 1500 pixels by 1200 pixels. Our goals were to present the images in their highest quality native colors and contrasts, to limit photographic artifact, and to highlight certain clinical features of the images with annotations or image insets. Every effort was made to maintain the integrity of the original photographs, with frequent reference to the original source. Image enhancement was reserved only for the selected image insets of this work, in cases where we felt particular features could be better illustrated with digital manipulation. We often magnified (though at no time was interpolation used to create new pixels) the insets, made them grayscale, and increased the contrast for the ease of the reader.

Ultimately, our intent is to present this color atlas and synopsis as an aid to the diagnosis and management of vitreoretinal diseases in the care of patients and as a resource for students of these conditions.

Mitchell C. Fineman, MD
Allen C. Ho, MD
Editors

Acknowledgments

Grateful acknowledgment is given to these consultants for their efforts and expertise in imaging and for their contributions to this publication:

Ms. Stefanie Carey, BS

Ms. Donna Galloway

Ms. Samantha Groch

Ms. MaryAnn Jay

Jay Klancnik, MD

Ms. Lisa Lavetsky

Henry C. Lee, MD

Ms. Elaine Liebenbaum, BS

Ms. Michele Skibo

Ms. Kristen Winkelspecht

Contents

Age-Related Macular Degeneration

Allen C. Ho ▪

Age-related macular degeneration (AMD) describes a common degenerative condition of the retina that may affect central vision. By definition, it occurs in individuals 50 years and older and is more prevalent with increasing age. Population-based surveys in the Western world vary but estimate the prevalence of AMD to be approximately 10% to 35% in individuals over the age of 50 years. AMD is divided into "dry" or nonexudative AMD and "wet" or exudative AMD.

DRY OR NONEXUDATIVE AGE-RELATED MACULAR DEGENERATION

Drusen are the clinical hallmark of dry AMD. They are subretinal pigment epithelial deposits between the basement membrane of the retinal pigment epithelium (RPE) and Bruch's membrane (Figs. 1-1 and 1-2) or within Bruch's membrane itself. Multiple types of drusen have been described, including large drusen (greater than 64 μm); small drusen

(63 μm or smaller); calcified drusen, which are yellow and glistening; and basal laminar drusen, which are small round diffuse drusen that are more apparent on fluorescein angiography than on clinical fundus examination (Fig. 1-3). Multiple large drusen are representative of a diffuse thickening of Bruch's membrane. Large drusen, also known as soft drusen, are a risk factor for more advanced AMD and vision loss. Small (also known as hard) drusen alone do not increase the risk for more advanced forms of AMD (Fig. 1-4).

Retinal pigment epithelial abnormalities, including nongeographic atrophy, focal hyperpigmentation, and frank geographic atrophy, are also common fundus features of dry AMD (Fig. 1-5). Granularity of the RPE may be an early feature of retinal pigment epithelial disturbance due to AMD. This may progress to areas of nongeographic atrophy (Fig. 1-6) in which there is loss of pigment of the RPE, but this is not discrete, and underlying choroidal vessels are not apparent. Geographic atrophy comprises discrete loss of RPE in a so-called cookie-cutter fashion with a minimal diameter of 250 μm

1

associated with underlying loss of choroidal stromal pigment and clearly visible underlying larger choroidal vessels (Fig. 1-7).

EPIDEMIOLOGY AND ETIOLOGY

- Drusen are seen increasingly with advancing age and typically are present in the sixth decade of life or later. Population-based studies estimate approximately 10% prevalence of early AMD (drusen) in the fifth decade of life, increasing to 35% in the seventh decade. Drusen may be seen in younger patients and may be heritable in these cases.

- The precise source of drusen material is not completely understood, but they are thought to represent degenerative products of retinal pigment epithelial cells; they are composed of lipids and glycoproteins, and may be mineralized. Retinal pigment epithelial alterations are seen increasingly with age and are common in the seventh, eighth, and ninth decades of life.

PATHOLOGY

- Transmission electron microscopy of eyes with drusen and dry AMD shows two types of deposits:

  - Basal laminar deposits consist of wide-spaced collagen localized between the retinal pigment epithelial plasma membrane and the retinal pigment epithelial basement membrane.

  - Basal linear deposits consist of lipid-rich material external to the basement membrane of the RPE in the inner collagenous zone of Bruch's membrane.

HISTORY

- Patients with drusen may be visually asymptomatic. Patients with multiple drusen

and associated retinal pigment epithelial abnormalities including granularity of the RPE, atrophy of the RPE, or focal hyperpigmentation will often note fluctuating vision, including central blurring. They typically will describe a need for increased light intensity in order to read and have difficulty adapting between different lighting.

- Patients with dry AMD and without evidence of geographic atrophy of the RPE or exudative AMD typically have good central vision between 20/20 and 20/60.

CLINICAL AND FLUORESCEIN ANGIOGRAPHIC SIGNS

- Fundus biomicroscopy shows subretinal pale yellow deposits that may vary in size from greater than 64 μm (large drusen) to small or hard drusen (63 μm or smaller) in diameter. Calcific drusen have a glistening appearance, and most patients with AMD have a mixture of clinical drusen types. Large drusen will often become confluent into larger drusenoid pigment epithelial detachments. Drusen should be considered fluid and dynamic structures that can appear or resolve over time (Fig. 1-8).

- An irregular granular appearance to the RPE is often seen in association with drusen. Areas of nongeographic atrophy or frank geographic atrophy are often appreciated after the spontaneous resolution of drusen and, in particular, drusenoid pigment epithelial detachments. Intraretinal pigment clumps or focal hyperpigmentation represents advanced retinal pigment epithelial degeneration as well.

- Fluorescein angiography typically demonstrates a patchy hyper- and hypofluorescence without leakage of dye. Drusen may show early or late hyperfluorescence, depending on the integrity of the overlying RPE and the histochemistry of the drusen themselves. Large soft drusen typically show early hypofluorescence and late hyperfluorescence (Fig. 1-9). This angiographic pattern is inconsistent, however, because some drusen, even those that are large, will show earlier hyperfluorescence (Fig. 1-10). Geographic atrophy shows discrete hyperfluorescence with stable boundaries throughout the angiogram (Fig. 1-11).

ASSOCIATED CLINICAL SIGNS

● When drusen are noted in patients over the age of 50, other features of AMD are often observed, including granularity and atrophy of the RPE. Drusen that are associated with subretinal fluid, hemorrhage, or lipid exudation due to choroidal neovascularization (CNV) are characteristics of exudative AMD.

DIFFERENTIAL DIAGNOSIS

● Drusen are subretinal and should be distinguished from intraretinal processes such as intraretinal lipid, retinal emboli, and cotton-wool spots. The borders of drusen may be more distinct in smaller hard drusen and less distinct with large drusen.

● Other yellow macular lesions can be included in the differential diagnosis of drusen, including the following:

  ▪ Pattern dystrophy: Presents in younger patients; lesions show geographic shape.

  ▪ Best's disease: Round or oval lesions may show different stages.

  ▪ Adult foveomacular dystrophy: Yellowish green subfoveal lesion; may simulate CNV on fluorescein angiography.

DIAGNOSTIC EVALUATION

● Patients with a sudden change in vision or new blur or distortion of central vision may be evaluated with fluorescein angiography to rule out exudative AMD.

● Careful fundus biomicroscopy is important to rule out subtle signs of exudative AMD.

● Optical coherence tomography (OCT) is an essential diagnostic tool in the evaluation of AMD patients and can help establish the presence of early exudative AMD and help determine the response to therapy.

PROGNOSIS AND MANAGEMENT

● Patients with drusen are counseled that they have the dry form of AMD and that most patients with drusen will not develop vision loss due to more advanced forms of AMD (exudative AMD and CNV or geographic atrophy). Patients with multiple large drusen are at a higher risk of developing CNV, particularly if the fellow eye has previously developed exudative AMD (Table 1-1). The 5-year risk of developing CNV in fellow eyes of patients with exudative AMD ranges between 40% and 85%. Management includes counseling regarding the importance of monitoring central vision in each eye with a test object such as the Amsler grid (Fig. 1-12).

TABLE 1-1. Risk of Choroidal Neovascularization (CNV) for Eyes with Drusen (Fellow Eye with Exudative CNV)

Overall estimate is 10% of patients per year with unilateral drusen will develop CNV. The Macular Photocoagulation Study Group has established risk factors that increase the risk of CNV:

Multiple large drusen

Focal hyperpigmentation

Hypertension

Smoking

- Information from the age-related eye disease study (AREDS) demonstrates that micronutrient and antioxidant supplementation (vitamin C, 500 mg; vitamin E, 400 IU; beta carotene, 15 mg; zinc, 80 mg as zinc oxide; and copper, 2 mg as cupric oxide) can effect a modest but definite reduction in clinical progression of AMD and moderate visual loss in patients with dry AMD and at least one large druse of 125 μm or larger. Data were not significant for patients with mild or borderline dry AMD (multiple small drusen or nonextensive intermediate drusen of 63 to 124 μm, pigment abnormalities, or any combination of these).

- Patients with focal hyperpigmentation have a higher risk of developing more advanced forms of AMD associated with vision loss and, in particular, CNV. Some believe that this clinical feature may represent a sign of early, ill-defined CNV in many cases. If there is a suspicion of early exudative AMD, then fluorescein angiography and OCT imaging may be performed. Since early retinal pigment epithelial abnormalities and granularity of the RPE may lead to nongeographic atrophy and frank geographic atrophy, they may be harbingers of vision loss.

- There are numerous clinical trials investigating potential therapies for dry AMD including other nutritional supplements such as omega 3 fatty acids, lutein and zeaxanthin carotenoids (AREDS 2 Study), visual cycle inhibitors, anti-inflammatory or complement inhibitors and stem cell therapies. An intraocular implantable telescope has been approved for patients with geographic atrophy based on clinical trial evidence.

FIGURE 1-1. **Large drusen. A.** Fundus photograph demonstrating predominantly large drusen, some of which are confluent (inset). Visual acuity was 20/25. **B** and **C.** Red free fundus image and OCT image of drusen at the level of Bruch's membrane and the retinal pigment epithelium. Note the irregular elevation of the retinal pigment epithelium caused by drusen.

FIGURE 1-2. **Confluent drusen.** Fundus photograph demonstrating multiple large, predominantly confluent drusen. Confluence is greatest temporal to the fovea. Confluent drusen are a risk factor for exudative age-related macular degeneration (AMD).

FIGURE 1-3. **Basal laminar drusen.** Fundus photograph demonstrating multiple small, round, diffuse drusen (inset) with large areas of confluence in the posterior pole and midperipheral retina. Basal laminar drusen may be more apparent with fluorescein angiography than clinically.

FIGURE 1-4. Hard drusen. Hard drusen (inset) are small (63 μm or smaller) and are not a risk factor for more advanced forms of AMD.

FIGURE 1-5. Focal hyperpigmentation. Fundus photograph showing multiple drusen with retinal pigment epithelial alterations (inset). Focal hyperpigmentation is noted in the fovea and just nasal to the fovea. Focal hyperpigmentation is a risk factor for more advanced forms of AMD associated with vision loss.

FIGURE 1-6. **Nongeographic atrophy. A.** Multiple large drusen are noted and there are areas of retinal pigment epithelial alterations. Surrounding the fovea superiorly and temporally are two areas of nongeographic atrophy. There is thinning of the retinal pigment epithelium (RPE), but the borders are not discrete around the entire lesion and the underlying larger choroidal vessels are not visible at this time. **B.** Fluorescein angiogram demonstrating transmission hyperfluorescence in nongeographic atrophy. Later images do not demonstrate leakage.

FIGURE 1-7. **End-stage geographic atrophy.** Large geographic atrophy involving the fovea. Note the visibility of the underlying larger choroidal vessels. Visual acuity was counting fingers.

FIGURE 1-8. **Drusenoid pigment epithelial detachment. A.** Right eye of a patient showing large confluent drusen in a drusenoid pigment epithelial detachment configuration. There is focal hyperpigmentation centered on the fovea. Visual acuity was 20/40. **B.** Left eye of the same patient showing spontaneous resolution of a drusenoid pigment epithelial detachment with a residual rim of confluent large drusen. Visual acuity was 20/30.

FIGURE 1-9. Multiple large drusen and confluent drusen. A. Drusen may spontaneously regress and progress to areas of right pigment epithelial atrophy (*arrow*). There is loss of foveal pigment from spontaneous resolution of drusen. **B.** Early-phase fluorescein angiogram demonstrating mild relative hypofluorescence corresponding to drusen (*arrow*).

(*continued*)

FIGURE 1-9. (*Continued*) **Multiple large drusen and confluent drusen. C.** Recirculation phase of fluorescein angiogram showing staining of drusen as discrete areas of hyperfluorescence (*arrow*).

FIGURE 1-10. **Multiple large drusen. A.** Multiple large confluent drusen (insets). Visual acuity was 20/25.

(*continued*)

FIGURE 1-10. (*Continued*) **Multiple large drusen. B.** Fluorescein angiogram showing early hyperfluorescence of the large drusen (*arrow*). **C.** Late fluorescein angiogram showing drusen staining but no evidence of choroidal neovascularization (CNV, *arrow*).

FIGURE 1-11. Atrophic AMD. A. Color fundus photograph demonstrating atrophic AMD. Multiple large- and medium-sized drusen are noted, and an area of geographic atrophy is noted just superior to the fovea (inset upper right). The borders are discrete, and the larger underlying choroidal vessels are visible. Areas of focal hyperpigmentation are noted as well (inset lower right). **B.** Early-phase fluorescein angiogram demonstrating transmission hyperfluorescence in the area of geographic atrophy.

(continued)

FIGURE 1-11. (*Continued*) **Atrophic AMD. C.** Recirculation phase photograph shows hyperfluorescence in the area of geographic atrophy but no evidence of leakage (inset). **D.** Late-phase fluorescein angiogram showing some fading of the choroidal fluorescence and staining hyperfluorescence in the region of geographic atrophy.

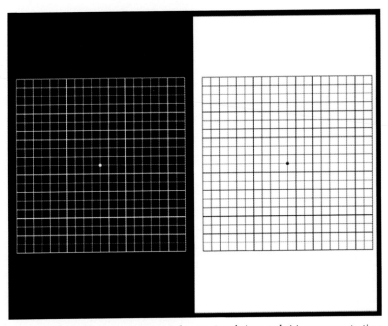

FIGURE 1-12. **Amsler grids.** Patients are instructed to monitor their central vision one eye at a time. Distortion, blurriness, or missing areas should prompt evaluation.

EXUDATIVE AGE-RELATED MACULAR DEGENERATION

Exudative AMD is characterized by intra-retinal, subretinal or subretinal pigment epithelial leakage, hemorrhage, or lipid exudation. CNV is the abnormal growth of new choroidal vessels into the subretinal space through defects in Bruch's membrane. In AMD, CNV may be invested within Bruch's membrane and the retinal pigment epithelium. Younger patients (non-AMD) who develop CNV typically develop this vascularization in the subretinal space alone. Pigment epithelial detachment describes a blister-like elevation of the retinal pigment epithelium and is another form of exudative AMD. Pigment epithelial detachments may be vascularized (fibrovascular pigment epithelial detachment) or may be purely serous and not associated with CNV. Disciform scarring is a final common pathway of CNV and pigment epithelial detachment in which there is progressive fibrosis and loss of macular photoreceptor function (Fig. 1-13).

Although the prevalence of the exudative form of AMD is low (approximately 10% of all patients with AMD), this form of late AMD accounts for the majority of legally blind patients with AMD (90%). The incidence of exudative AMD is on the rise, with an estimated 200,000 individuals experiencing severe central loss of vision due to exudative AMD in the year 2011. This is expected to rise to approximately 500,000 per year by the year 2030.

EPIDEMIOLOGY AND ETIOLOGY

- CNV is the leading cause of central blindness among the elderly in the United States and in most of the Western world. The pathophysiology of exudative AMD and the specific stimuli required for the development of CNV are not well understood.

PATHOLOGY

- CNV is typically derived from choroidal venules and may invade above and beneath the RPE through breaks in Bruch's membrane.

HISTORY

- Patients with exudative AMD may note loss of vision, distortion of vision, or blurring of vision. Early changes may be more evident with Amsler grid monitoring.

- Patients may be asymptomatic, however, if the fellow eye continues to function well.

- There may be a history of loss of vision in the fellow eye due to exudative AMD.

CLINICAL OCT AND FLUORESCEIN ANGIOGRAPHIC SIGNS

- Careful slit lamp fundus biomicroscopy is important in the diagnosis of exudative AMD. Clinical signs of retinal edema, subretinal fluid, lipid exudation and intra and subretinal hemorrhage can be subtle. In particular, it is difficult to determine retinal fluid when there are areas of RPE depigmentation or atrophy.

- OCT imaging of exudative AMD may reveal thickening of the macula or retinal pigment epithelium. There is often intraretinal cystic change, subretinal fluid or RPE detachment. Quantitative imaging over time and with image registration affords information to determine response to therapy. Not all cystic change may represent true edema as chronic retinal fluid may create tubular changes that mimic edema.

- Fluorescein angiographic classification of exudative AMD was particularly important prior to pharmacologic therapy, specifically anti-vascular endothelial growth factor treatment.

Classic Choroidal Neovascularization

- Fundus biomicroscopy may reveal a greenish gray subretinal lesion often with associated submacular fluid, hemorrhage, or lipid exudation due to the incompetent vasculature of the CNV. Occasionally, a ring of dark pigment may surround the CNV. The pigment ring is more commonly observed in patients with classic CNV. Fluorescein angiography is necessary to characterize the nature and location of the CNV. CNV may be subfoveal if localized beneath the geometric center of the fovea, juxtafoveal if localized from 1 to 199 μm from the foveal center, or extrafoveal if 200 μm or farther from the center of the fovea.

- Classic CNV is characterized by early appearance of fluorescein leakage during the choroidal and retinal vascular filling phases of the fluorescein angiogram (Fig. 1-14). The leakage may be characterized by a lacy appearance of a network of blood vessels (but this is not requisite) and typically is fairly well delineated. More importantly, the lesion must demonstrate continued leakage through the recirculation and late phases of the fluorescein angiogram.

Occult Choroidal Neovascularization

- Fundus biomicroscopy may demonstrate irregular elevation of the RPE most commonly in association with submacular fluid, hemorrhage, or lipid exudation due to the incompetent vasculature of the CNV; less commonly, irregular elevation of the RPE alone may comprise the only clinical sign of occult CNV. Occult CNV is characterized by later appearing and less intense fluorescein angiographic leakage.

- One type of occult CNV, fibrovascular pigment epithelial detachment, is characterized by irregular stippled hyperfluorescence with mild leakage or staining of fluorescein dye in poorly demarcated boundaries of leakage (Fig. 1-15). The second type of occult CNV,

late leakage of undetermined source, is characterized by leakage of fluorescein dye in the recirculation phase of the fluorescein angiogram associated with pooling of fluorescein dye in the subretinal space and areas of speckled hyperfluorescence (Fig. 1-16).

- Most patients with exudative AMD demonstrate a combination of classic and occult CNV (Fig. 1-17). Characterization of the different types of CNV is important as management recommendations are based not only on the location of the lesion, but also on the nature of the CNV.

Fibrovascular Pigment Epithelial Detachment and Serous Pigment Epithelial Detachment

- Fibrovascular pigment epithelial detachment is a form of occult CNV. Purely serous pigment epithelial detachment is characterized by a blister-like elevation of sub-RPE fluid. Fundus biomicroscopy shows an orange ring that illuminates with a slit-lamp light beam. A serous pigment epithelial detachment is often associated with a serous detachment of the neurosensory macula as well. Fluorescein angiography shows a uniform rapid filling of fluorescein dye beneath the boundaries of the pigment epithelial detachment (Fig. 1-18).

- Fibrovascular pigment epithelial detachments may have associated serous retinal pigment epithelial detachments and are often denoted by a notch on the fluorescein angiogram (Fig. 1-19A, B). The notch represents the CNV. Fibrovascular pigment epithelial detachments are more likely to have a serosanguineous component in the sub-RPE fluid, and this may be visualized ophthalmoscopically. Indocyanine green angiography may be helpful in imaging presumed CNV in the setting of occult CNV and pigment epithelial detachment (Fig. 1-19C, D).

Retinal Pigment Epithelial Tears

- Retinal pigment epithelial tears may be observed in association with pigment epithelial detachments. A scrolled edge of RPE may be apparent with fundus biomicroscopy and sometimes is associated with a flattening of the retinal pigment epithelial detachment. Vision loss is typically observed with a retinal pigment epithelial tear, although in some cases, good central vision is preserved in the short term. Fluorescein angiography shows early intense hyperfluorescence corresponding to the area of denuded RPE and relative hypofluorescence where there is scrolled and redundant retinal pigment epithelial tissue (Fig. 1-20).

Submacular Hemorrhage

- A large submacular hemorrhage may be associated with apoplectic loss of central vision. It may be the presenting manifestation of exudative AMD or may follow the development of classic or occult CNV, or both (Fig. 1-21).

- Fundus biomicroscopy shows subretinal and sometimes preretinal or subretinal pigment epithelial hemorrhage that may have significant elevation greater than 1 mm in height. The extent of the hemorrhage may be limited or sometimes can extend to involve the entire posterior pole or beyond. Vision loss typically correlates with the extent of subfoveal involvement and the two-dimensional size of the submacular hemorrhage.

- Fluorescein angiography may or may not show source CNV. The submacular hemorrhage will typically obscure underlying normal and pathologic choroidal fluorescence.

Disciform Scar

- Disciform scar is the final common pathway of exudative AMD. Thin or thick fibrotic submacular scarring may be observed, and there may be associated chronic submacular fluid, lipid exudation, cystoid macular edema, and submacular hemorrhage (see Fig. 1-13).

Occasionally, retinochoroidal anastomoses are seen connecting the underlying pathologic CNV and fibrosis with the retinal circulation. Fluorescein angiography shows staining of the disciform scar and leakage from any residual active CNV.

DIFFERENTIAL DIAGNOSIS

- Signs of exudative AMD such as retinal hemorrhage, lipid exudation, macular edema, and submacular fluid may be confused with non-AMD conditions. For example, serous detachments of the macula may be associated with central serous retinopathy, although this is typically seen in younger patients.

- Intraretinal hemorrhage can be seen in retinal venous occlusive disease, hypertensive retinopathy, or diabetic retinopathy, but it also may be the presenting sign of early CNV.

- Cystoid macular edema may be a presenting sign of CNV. Cystoid macular edema due to CNV may be confused with pseudophakic cystoid macular edema. Macular edema associated with retinal vascular conditions such as venous occlusive disease, parafoveal telangiectasia, or diabetic retinopathy may present in similar fashion to exudative AMD. Stereoscopic fluorescein angiography is critical to make the correct diagnosis.

- Polypoidal choroidal vasculopathy is an exudative maculopathy that may be seen in all races but usually is observed in African Americans or Asian Americans in whom exudative AMD is less common. This condition is characterized by choroidal aneurysms with associated serosanguineous pigment epithelial detachments and submacular exudation. This particular condition is imaged well with indocyanine green angiography, whereby choroidal saccular aneurysms may be highlighted in a peripapillary distribution or in a macular distribution.

- Large submacular or intraretinal hemorrhages can be seen in the setting of trauma, choroidal tumor, or retinal arterial macroaneurysm, and these conditions, in addition to exudative AMD, should be considered in the context of this clinical presentation.

PROGNOSIS AND MANAGEMENT

- The central visual prognosis of exudative AMD has dramatically improved with the advent of anti-VEGF injection therapies; peripheral vision typically remains unaffected. Over 90% of patients can experience maintenance of vision over time with frequent anti-VEGF injections. Up to a third or higher of these patients can experience significant visual gains with this treatment. There are a variety of clinical research trials investigating new treatments for exudative AMD.

Evidence-based and Other Therapies

- The current benchmark foundation therapy for exudative AMD is monthly (ranibizumab, Lucentis) to bimonthly (aflibercept, Eylea) anti-VEGF injections as established by randomized controlled clinical trials that frequent monitoring visits and frequent injections afford the highest chance of best visual acuity.

- Ranibizumab, aflibercept and off-label bevacizumab appear to have greater potency compared with pegaptanib (Macugen) although a comparative trial has not been performed. Currently, there are multiple clinical trials exploring the potential enhanced efficacy of combining anti-VEGF injection therapy with other pharmacologic agents.

- **Thermal laser photocoagulation:** In the 1980s the Macular Photocoagulation Study

Group Classic established that thermal laser photocoagulation was the treatment of choice for well-delineated extrafoveal CNV. The major problem with this therapy is that up to 60% of eyes will develop recurrent CNVs, the majority of which are subfoveal (Fig. 1-22). Currently, many specialists would choose anti-VEGF injection therapy for extrafoveal CNV because it is less destructive and potentially more efficacious.

- **Verteporfin photodynamic therapy (PDT):** Prior to anti-VEGF injection therapy the Treatment of AMD with Photodynamic Therapy Study Group established that verteporfin PDT was the treatment of choice for predominantly classic subfoveal CNV. Although visual improvement was achieved in only a minority of eyes (approximately 15% at 1 year), treated eyes show more visual stability than observed eyes over 2 years. Treatment benefit was also established for occult CNV but not for mixed lesions that are less than predominantly classic CNV (Fig. 1-23). Currently, verteporfin PDT is generally considered as a potential adjunctive treatment for exudative AMD and is often performed at reduced energy fluence. PDT may play a larger role in the treatment of polypoidal choroidal vasculopathy compared with exudative AMD.

Surgical Therapies

- The submacular surgery trials did not demonstrate benefit for surgical evacuation of large submacular hemorrhage and CNV. Surgical displacement of large submacular hemorrhages with or without clot lysing agents such as tissue plasminogen activator may improve vision for some patients and may also reveal underlying CNV—at this time there are no surgical clinical trials exploring the displacement of large submacular hemorrhage.

FIGURE 1-13. **Disciform scar.** A large area of submacular fibrosis with chronic submacular fluid is noted. Disciform scarring is the final common pathway for exudative AMD. Visual acuity is counting fingers eccentrically.

FIGURE 1-14. **Exudative AMD, classic CNV. A.** Shallow submacular fluid and intraretinal hemorrhage are noted.

(*continued*)

FIGURE 1-14. (*Continued*) **Exudative AMD, classic CNV. B.** Arterio-venous phase fluorescein angiogram showing a cartwheel of extrafoveal classic CNV (*arrow*) and hypofluorescence corresponding to retinal hemorrhage. **C.** Recirculation phase photograph showing early leakage of dye from the classic CNV.

(*continued*)

FIGURE 1-14. (*Continued*) **Exudative AMD, classic CNV. D.** Late image showing some pooling of dye beneath the neurosensory retina. **E.** Thermal laser photocoagulation is performed and shows retinal whitening.

(*continued*)

FIGURE 1-14. (*Continued*) **Exudative AMD, classic CNV. F.** Three weeks later there is evidence of atrophy in the area of laser treatment and resolution of the submacular fluid. **G.** Fluorescein angiogram showing no evidence of recurrent CNV at 3 weeks. The patient remains at risk for the subsequent development of recurrent CNV.

FIGURE 1-15. Occult CNV. A. Color fundus photograph demonstrating drusen and slightly turbid submacular fluid centered inferior to the fovea (inset). **B.** Recirculation phase fluorescein angiogram demonstrating ill-defined stippled hyperfluorescence inferior to the fovea. There is some drusen staining as well (inset).

(*continued*)

FIGURE 1-15. (*Continued*) **Occult CNV. C.** Fluorescein angiogram demonstrating some mild leakage of fluorescein dye beneath the fovea. Late fluorescein angiographic images show ill-defined leakage inferior to the fovea (inset). **D.** Red-free image of occult CNV. **E.** OCT image demonstrating intraretinal fluid, subretinal fluid and retinal pigment epithelial detachment.

FIGURE 1-16. Occult CNV. A. Color fundus photograph showing turbid submacular fluid and drusen (*arrow*). **B.** Fluorescein angiogram showing ill-defined stippled hyperfluorescence temporal to the fovea (*arrow*).

(*continued*)

FIGURE 1-16. (*Continued*) **Occult CNV. C.** Fluorescein angiogram showing more diffuse ill-defined leakage (*arrow*). **D.** Late fluorescein angiogram showing poorly demarcated, stippled hyperfluorescence and leakage of dye characteristic of occult CNV (*arrow*).

FIGURE 1-17. Classic and occult CNV. A. Fundus photograph demonstrating macular edema as well as shallow submacular fluid due to exudative AMD (*arrow*). Some drusen are noted peripheral to the neurosensory detachment. **B.** Arterio-venous phase fluorescein angiogram showing hyperfluorescence consistent with combination of classic and occult CNV. Classic component is superior and temporal.

(*continued*)

FIGURE 1-17. (*Continued*) **Classic and occult CNV. C.** Midphase fluorescein angiogram demonstrating leakage from the subfoveal CNV. Classic component shows brighter hyperfluorescence than the occult CNV. **D.** Pooling of fluorescein dye below the neurosensory detachment from classic and occult CNV (inset).

FIGURE 1-18. Retinal pigment epithelial detachment. A. Color fundus photograph showing a retinal pigment epithelial detachment with submacular fluid centered temporal to the fovea. Some drusen are noted temporal to the detachment. **B.** Midphase fluorescein angiogram showing hyperfluorescence corresponding to a large retinal pigment epithelial detachment.

(*continued*)

FIGURE 1-18. (*Continued*) **Retinal pigment epithelial detachment. C.** Recirculation phase fluorescein angiogram demonstrating pooling of dye beneath the pigment epithelial detachment and a fibrovascular component centered on the fovea. **D.** Fluorescein angiogram showing the extent of the serous and fibrovascular pigment epithelial detachment. The area of involvement remains unchanged from the recirculation phase image.

(*continued*)

FIGURE 1-18. (*Continued*) **Retinal pigment epithelial detachment. E.** Red-free fundus image of retinal pigment epithelial detachment. **F.** OCT image demonstrates retinal pigment epithelial detachment and associated macular edema.

FIGURE 1-19. **Serous pigment epithelial detachment. A.** Color fundus photograph demonstrating a blister-like elevation of a serous pigment epithelial detachment (inset). **B.** Fluorescein angiogram showing a serous pigment epithelium detachment centered on the fovea with a notch on the nasal border. The notch may represent an area of CNV.

(continued)

FIGURE 1-19. (*Continued*) **Serous pigment epithelial detachment. C.** Another patient with pigment epithelial detachment seen on fluorescein angiography; no notch is observed. **D.** Indocyanine green angiogram showing a focal area of hyperfluorescence (*arrow*) within the pigment epithelial detachment corresponding to presumed CNV.

FIGURE 1-20. **Retinal pigment epithelial tear. A.** A retinal pigment epithelial tear is noted by the discrete borders of the loss of pigment in the temporal macula. A scrolled edge can be seen as a curved hyperpigmented line extending through the fovea (inset). **B.** Early-phase fluorescein angiogram showing a bright, well-delineated area of hyperfluorescence corresponding to the retinal pigment epithelial tear. The redundant scrolled edge of the tear shows as relative hypofluorescence in an arc through the fovea (inset).

(*continued*)

FIGURE 1-20. (*Continued*) **Retinal pigment epithelial tear. C.** Late-phase fluorescein angiogram showing no evidence of fluorescein dye leakage beyond the temporal border of the tear (inset). **D.** Thirty months later, the color fundus photograph shows some submacular fibrosis and atrophy in the retinal pigment epithelial tear. Underlying choroidal vessels are visible in the region of the tear (inset).

FIGURE 1-21. Submacular hemorrhage. Submacular hemorrhage can cause dramatic sudden loss of central vision in patients with exudative AMD. Note that some overlying retinal vessels are visible, the clue that the hemorrhage is subretinal.

FIGURE 1-22. Recurrent CNV after thermal laser treatment. A. Color fundus photograph shows prior area of hyperpigmented thermal laser photocoagulation scar and new submacular hemorrhage and fluid extending through the fovea. **B.** Fluorescein angiogram showing the hyperfluorescent, subfoveal, recurrent CNV surrounded by a rim of hypofluorescence. The old thermal laser scar is predominantly hypofluorescent inferior to the CNV.

FIGURE 1-23. **Anti-VEGF therapy for exudative AMD. A.** Color fundus photograph demonstrating serous macular detachment and retinal hemorrhage prior to treatment with monthly intravitreal ranibizumab anti-VEGF therapy. Visual acuity was 20/100. **B.** Pretreatment fluorescein angiogram demonstrating occult subfoveal CNV.

(continued)

FIGURE 1-23. (*Continued*) **Anti-VEGF therapy for exudative AMD. C.** Pretreatment fluorescein angiogram demonstrating leakage within the neurosensory detachment. **D.** Pretreatment OCT image demonstrates CNV and thickening of the macula.

(*continued*)

FIGURE 1-23. (*Continued*) **Anti-VEGF therapy for exudative AMD. E.** One year posttreatment color fundus photograph reveals diminished submacular fluid and absence of retinal hemorrhage. Visual acuity was 20/40. **F and G.** Posttreatment fluorescein angiogram demonstrating less leakage and staining.

(continued)

FIGURE 1-23. (*Continued*) **Anti-VEGF therapy for exudative AMD. H.** Posttreatment OCT image reveals reduced macular thickening. Visual acuity was 20/40.

2

Macular Diseases

Nikolas J.S. London and Mitchell S. Fineman

MACULAR EPIRETINAL MEMBRANE

Macular epiretinal membrane is an acquired formation of a semitransparent fibrocellular membrane in the macula.

EPIDEMIOLOGY AND ETIOLOGY

- Macular epiretinal membranes may be either idiopathic or secondary to other intraocular abnormalities, including retinal breaks, retinal vascular disease, uveitis, blunt and penetrating trauma, and surgery. Idiopathic macular epiretinal membranes are most common after 50 years of age.

- Males and females are affected equally.

- Bilateral macular epiretinal membranes occur in approximately 20% of patients, with the severity of the membranes usually asymmetric.

- Most patients have posterior vitreous detachment (PVD), and it is thought that this phenomenon may contribute to formation of the membrane. After PVD, a portion of posterior cortical vitreous may be left behind on the macula, or the internal limiting membrane may be disrupted, allowing glial cells to proliferate on the surface of the retina. These proliferating glial cells form the epiretinal membrane. After retinal break formation and trauma, retinal pigment epithelial cells may escape into the vitreous cavity and settle upon the macula. These cells may then undergo metaplasia to glial cells, allowing the formation of macular epiretinal membranes.

HISTORY

- If the macular epiretinal membrane is thin and not producing distortion of the retina, then the patient is usually asymptomatic. With progressive thickening and contraction of the membrane, patients begin to notice decreased vision, metamorphopsia, and macropsia or micropsia.

- Most patients maintain vision better than 20/50.

- Most epiretinal membranes progress slowly and occasionally improve spontaneously.

IMPORTANT CLINICAL SIGNS

- Macular epiretinal membranes initially appear as translucent, glistening membranes over, or adjacent to, the central macula (Fig. 2-1). There may be a "pseudohole" appearance over the fovea. As the membrane matures, it becomes more opaque (Fig. 2-2A).

- There may be associated superficial hemorrhages or nerve fiber layer infarcts.

- The membranes contract centrally and cause wrinkling and distortion of the underlying retina. This wrinkling and distortion gives rise to other names for this condition: cellophane maculopathy, surface wrinkling retinopathy, and macular pucker. If the distortion is severe, cystoid macular edema and even shallow tractional retinal detachment can occur.

DIFFERENTIAL DIAGNOSIS

- Cystoid macular edema
- Choroidal neovascularization (CNV)
- Macular hole
- Choroidal folds
- Combined hamartoma of the retina
- Retinal pigment epithelium

DIAGNOSTIC EVALUATION

- Usually measurement of visual acuity, Amsler grid testing (to assess for metamorphopsia, macropsia, or micropsia) and ophthalmoscopy suffice to make the diagnosis of macular epiretinal membrane. Slit-lamp biomicroscopy with either a noncontact or a contact lens greatly facilitates diagnosis.

- Optical coherence tomography (OCT) has become standard in documenting the presence of an epiretinal membrane. OCT reveals a hyperreflective band on the surface of the retina, associated with retinal distortion, thickening, and/or cystoid edema in advanced cases.

- Fluorescein angiography will clearly delineate retinal vascular distortion and leakage that may occur from cystoid macular edema (Fig. 2-2B, C).

PROGNOSIS AND MANAGEMENT

- Most patients with uniocular macular epiretinal membrane and vision better than 20/50 are usually not significantly symptomatic and do not require intervention. Patients with vision of 20/60 or worse and those patients with intolerable distortion may benefit from pars plana vitrectomy with membrane peeling and removal (Fig. 2-3).

- Rarely, the membrane may spontaneously release, leading to resolution of symptoms.

FIGURE 2-1. Macular epiretinal membrane. Glistening membrane over the macula causing distortion of central retina.

FIGURE 2-2. Macular epiretinal membrane. A. Thick membrane over the macula causing distortion of the central retina.

(continued)

FIGURE 2-2. (*Continued*) **Macular epiretinal membrane. B.** Fluorescein angiogram showing distortion of the macular retina. **C.** Late-phase fluorescein angiogram showing intraretinal leakage of dye from distorted retinal vessels.

FIGURE 2-3. Macular epiretinal membrane. A. Preoperative appearance of membrane (inset); visual acuity was 6/60. Note the retinal folds and retinal vascular compression and tortuosity. **B.** Postoperative appearance of membrane (inset); visual acuity was 6/12. There is less retinal vascular tortuosity.

IDIOPATHIC MACULAR HOLE

I diopathic macular hole is an acquired full-thickness defect of retina in the central macula.

EPIDEMIOLOGY AND ETIOLOGY

- Idiopathic macular holes typically occur in the sixth through eighth decades of life with a 3:1 predominance in women.

- The incidence of bilaterality is 5% to 10%.

- Tangential vitreoretinal traction is the presumed cause of development of idiopathic macular hole.

- The Gass classification of the stages of idiopathic macular hole development is helpful in understanding the progression of the disease and the biomicroscopic findings (**Table 2-1**).

- Patients with a full-thickness macular hole in one eye and an impending macular hole with no PVD in the fellow eye are at substantial risk of progression to stage 2 macular hole in

the second eye. Patients with a full-thickness macular hole in one eye and a normal retina with PVD in the fellow eye are at very little risk of progressing to macular hole in the second eye.

HISTORY

- Patients usually report decreased visual acuity with central scotoma. There may be metamorphopsia.

- Often patients notice decreased vision in the affected eye when the fellow eye is incidentally covered as for a routine eye examination.

IMPORTANT CLINICAL SIGNS

- Depending on the stage and severity of the macular hole, the visual acuity may be near normal or severely reduced to less than 20/400.

- Amsler grid testing will often reveal metamorphopsia or a central scotoma. Ophthalmoscopy and slit-lamp biomicroscopy reveal findings consistent with the stage of the macular hole.

TABLE 2-1. Stages of Development of Idiopathic Macular Hole

Stage 1A	Early contraction of outer part of vitreous cortex with foveolar detachment (impending macular hole)
Stage 1B	Further vitreous contraction and condensation of the prefoveal vitreous cortex with foveal detachment (impending macular hole)
Stage 2	Small (<400 μm) perifoveal dehiscence
Stage 3	Larger (>400 μm) central full-thickness hole usually accompanied by a rim of retinal elevation; the posterior cortical vitreous remains attached; there may be a small operculum overlying the macular hole
Stage 4	Macular hole has an associated complete posterior vitreous detachment; these holes are usually large (>400 μm).

Based on Gass JD. Reappraisal of biomicroscopic classification of stages of development of a macular hole. *Am J Opthalmol.* 1995;119:752–759.

■ Stage 1 holes appear as a small yellow cyst or ring around the fovea with a loss of the foveal depression (Fig. 2-4).

■ Stage 2 holes appear as a small round or crescent-shaped defect in the fovea (Fig. 2-5).

■ Stage 3 holes have a dark round defect in the fovea, often with a cuff of subretinal fluid accumulation (Fig. 2-6).

■ Stage 4 holes are often larger than stage 3 holes and are associated with a PVD (Fig. 2-7).

● There are often small yellow dots in the center of the hole at the level of the retinal pigment epithelium (Fig. 2-8).

ASSOCIATED CLINICAL SIGNS

● The Watzke–Allen sign is the patient's description of discontinuance in the center of a thin slit beam shone over the fovea.

DIFFERENTIAL DIAGNOSIS

● Macular epiretinal membrane with pseudohole
● Cystoid macular edema
● Central serous retinopathy (CSR)
● Choroidal neovascular membrane
● Solar retinopathy
● Adult vitelliform dystrophy

DIAGNOSTIC EVALUATION

● Clinical examination alone is often diagnostic. Fluorescein angiography in eyes with stage 2, 3, or 4 macular holes will reveal early central hyperfluorescence in the fovea corresponding to loss of xanthophyll pigment and retinal pigment epithelial depigmentation and atrophy at the base of the hole. OCT clearly distinguishes between partial- and full-thickness holes. (Fig. 2-9).

PROGNOSIS AND MANAGEMENT

● No treatment is recommended for stage 1 macular holes because these resolve spontaneously in 50% of cases. Spontaneous resolution of more advanced stages of macular hole can occur, but it is rare.

● Vitrectomy can be performed for more advanced stages of macular hole. The surgery consists of a standard pars plana vitrectomy, peeling of the posterior hyaloid, and injection of a long-acting gas such as perfluoropropane. Peeling of the internal membrane may also be done. Patients must then maintain face-down positioning for 1 to 2 weeks to allow the gas bubble to tamponade the hole. Recent evidence suggests that face-down positioning is not as critical as once believed, but this needs to be studied further. The success rate for macular hole surgery approaches 80% to 90% with closure of the hole and improvement in visual acuity (Fig. 2-10).

● Negative prognostic indicators include a long duration of hole presence (i.e. greater than 1 year) and larger size of the hole.

FIGURE 2-4. Idiopathic macular hole, stage 1. A. Stage 1 macular hole with yellow ring appearance around the fovea. Visual acuity remains 6/7.5. **B.** Optical coherence tomography showing stage 1 macular hole.

FIGURE 2-5. **Idiopathic macular hole, stage 2. A.** Stage 2 macular hole appears as a small round defect in the fovea (inset). **B.** Optical coherence tomography showing stage 2 macular hole with persistent traction on one edge of the hole.

FIGURE 2-6. **Idiopathic macular hole, stage 3. A.** Stage 3 macular hole with cuff of subretinal fluid around the hole. **B.** Optical coherence tomography showing stage 3 macular hole.

FIGURE 2-7. Idiopathic macular hole, stage 4. A. Stage 4 macular hole; note condensed vitreous of posterior vitreous detachment overlying inferotemporal vascular arcade (*arrow*). **B.** Optical coherence tomography showing stage 4 macular hole.

FIGURE 2-8. Idiopathic macular hole, chronic. A. Chronic stage 4 macular hole with subretinal precipitates (inset). **B.** Retinal pigment epithelial ring around macular hole indicates chronicity.

FIGURE 2-9. **Idiopathic macular hole.** Optical coherence tomography (OCT) of stage 4 macular hole showing complete defect in retina.

FIGURE 2-10. Idiopathic macular hole. A. Preoperative appearance of stage 3 macular hole (yellow spots are incidental drusen). **B.** Postoperative appearance of stage 3 macular hole; note closed appearance of hole. Vision improved to 6/12 from 6/30.

VITREOMACULAR TRACTION SYNDROME

Vitreomacular traction syndrome (VMTS) is an acquired condition in which there is partial separation of the posterior hyaloid with persistent attachment to the macula and, occasionally, the optic nerve head.

EPIDEMIOLOGY AND ETIOLOGY

- VMTS occurs in the same age group as those who develop PVD. PVD is uncommon before 50 years of age and is present in over 50% of people aged 70 years and older.

HISTORY

- Patients who have VMTS experience progressive distortion and visual loss, which is often more severe than that occurring with macular epiretinal membrane.

IMPORTANT CLINICAL SIGNS

- The posterior hyaloid is visibly thickened. There is macular distortion, often with tractional retinal detachment in the macula. Retinal striae may be present. There may be traction in the peripapillary region. An epiretinal membrane may be seen clinically (**Fig. 2-11**).

DIFFERENTIAL DIAGNOSIS

- Macular epiretinal membrane
- Combined hamartoma of the retina and retinal pigment epithelium

DIAGNOSTIC EVALUATION

- Fluorescein angiography may reveal retinal vascular distortion and leakage. There may be cystoid macular edema and optic nerve edema.
- Spectral-domain OCT helps determine the presence of VMTS as well as associated macular edema and tractional detachment.

PROGNOSIS AND MANAGEMENT

- Occasionally patients may experience spontaneous improvement if PVD occurs.
- Surgical intervention is indicated if visual acuity is reduced to 20/70 or worse. During vitrectomy surgery, the posterior hyaloid is removed, as are any epiretinal membranes in the macular region. The retinal architecture can be restored to a normal appearance. The vision can be improved but usually complete recovery does not occur due to residual macular edema.
- Pharmacologic vitreolysis with microplasmin is currently under investigation for the treatment of VMTS, with promising initial results.

FIGURE 2-11. Vitreomacular traction syndrome. A. Adhesion of the vitreous to a premacular membrane elevates the fovea and creates macular distortion. **B.** OCT showing vitreomacular traction. **C.** Severe vitreomacular traction may lead to secondary macular hole formation.

CYSTOID MACULAR EDEMA

Cystoid macular edema (CME) is the result of accumulation of intraretinal fluid in the perifoveal region. Fluid accumulates in cystic spaces that may be visible clinically and on fluorescein angiography.

EPIDEMIOLOGY AND ETIOLOGY

• CME is most commonly seen after cataract surgery. Other types of ocular surgery, such as trabeculectomy, laser photocoagulation and cryoretinopexy, may also give rise to CME.

• Less commonly, CME is seen in association with diabetic retinopathy, CNV, uveitis, retinal vein obstruction, perifoveal telangiectasis, retinitis pigmentosa, and other entities.

HISTORY

• CME following cataract surgery typically has its onset 6 to 10 weeks after surgery. Patients experience an initial improvement in vision only to be followed by decreasing central vision in the range of 6/40 to 6/100.

IMPORTANT CLINICAL SIGNS

• When CME is present in the post–cataract surgery patient, there is often no abnormality noted in the anterior segment.

• On slit-lamp biomicroscopy, patients will have cystic spaces in the perifoveal area (Fig. 2-12A), best seen by narrowing the slit beam adjacent to the fovea. There will also be thickening of the central macula and, occasionally, tiny round intraretinal hemorrhages at the edge of the foveal avascular zone.

ASSOCIATED CLINICAL SIGNS

• There may be no associated clinical signs when CME occurs after cataract surgery. However, CME is more common after complicated cataract surgery in which there has been rupture of the posterior capsule and vitreous loss. Such findings as vitreous to the wound, iris to the wound, iris atrophy, and an opening in the posterior capsule may therefore be present.

• When CME is present in association with other ophthalmic diseases, then the findings of those entities will be present. For example, pigment migration into the retinal midperiphery will be present in patients with CME in association with retinitis pigmentosa, and diffuse intraretinal hemorrhages will be present in patients with CME in association with retinal venous occlusive disease.

DIFFERENTIAL DIAGNOSIS

• CNV
• Diabetic macular edema

DIAGNOSTIC EVALUATION

• Fluorescein angiography is helpful in establishing the diagnosis of CME. Fluorescein angiography shows accumulation of dye in the perifoveal region in a petalloid pattern (Fig. 2-12B). There is often leakage of dye from the optic nerve head (Fig. 2-12C), often called Irvine–Gass syndrome. The foveal avascular zone is not enlarged in uncomplicated CME.

• Angiographic CME may be present in as many as 60% of patients following routine cataract surgery. Clinically significant CME, in which patients are symptomatic, occurs in 2% to 10% of patients following uncomplicated cataract surgery.

PROGNOSIS AND MANAGEMENT

• Most patients who suffer postoperative CME will undergo spontaneous resolution within 6 months. Therapeutic intervention is indicated if patients are symptomatic with decreased vision.

• There is no single accepted regimen for management of postoperative CME. The most common therapies are topical or periocular corticosteroids, topical nonsteroidal anti-inflammatory drugs (NSAIDs), and oral carbonic anhydrase inhibitors in various frequencies of administration and combination of agents. A typical starting regimen is topical prednisolone acetate and a topical NSAID 4 times daily for several months. For unresponsive cases, periocular or intravitreal corticosteroid injection can be considered. Alternatively, intravitreal anti-VEGF or low-dose systemic acetazolamide can be considered.

• Surgical intervention with Nd:YAG laser vitreolysis for thin strands of vitreous trapped in the cataract wound or vitrectomy for more extensive vitreous or iris incarceration or vitreomacular adhesion may result in resolution of CME.

FIGURE 2-12. Cystoid macular edema. A. The normal foveal reflex is lost and there are cystoid changes in the central macula. **B.** Early arteriovenous transit phase fluorescein angiogram showing leakage of dye in the perifoveal area.

(continued)

FIGURE 2-12. (*Continued*) **Cystoid macular edema. C.** Late-phase fluorescein angiogram showing "petalloid" pattern of dye leakage in addition to leakage of dye from the optic nerve head. **D.** OCT showing cystoid macular edema.

POLYPOIDAL CHOROIDAL VASCULOPATHY

Polypoidal choroidal vasculopathy (PCV) is an idiopathic hemorrhagic disorder of the macula.

EPIDEMIOLOGY AND ETIOLOGY

- PCV is a disorder of the inner choroidal vasculature in which there is a network of branching vessels deep to the choriocapillaris in association with terminal aneurysmal dilations. It is assumed that PCV represents a form of CNV. However, polypoidal CNV behaves differently from other forms of CNV, and the visual prognosis is better compared with CNV.
- PCV was initially described in elderly black women but is now known to occur in all races with preponderance in heavily pigmented individuals.
- Men are equally affected as women.
- The average age of onset of polypoidal CNV is much younger than that of age-related macular degeneration, but the range of age at onset is wider (less than 25 to more than 85 years). Lesions are usually bilateral, but patients have been followed for years with unilateral involvement.

HISTORY

- Patients with PCV present with decreased and distorted vision if serosanguineous complications occur in the macula.

IMPORTANT CLINICAL SIGNS

- Patients with PCV may develop chronic recurrent acute serosanguineous detachments of the retina and retinal pigment epithelium. The vascular lesions may be seen with slit-lamp biomicroscopy as reddish orange spheroidal or polypoidal lesions. The lesions have a predilection for the peripapillary area but may be seen elsewhere in the macula and even in the periphery.
- Rarely, bullous or total serosanguineous retinal detachment with or without vitreous hemorrhage may occur.

ASSOCIATED CLINICAL SIGNS

- Systemic hypertension is often associated with severe PCV with visual loss.

DIFFERENTIAL DIAGNOSIS

- Age-related macular degeneration with CNV
- Central serous choroidopathy
- Retinal pigment epithelial detachment

DIAGNOSTIC EVALUATION

- Serosanguineous detachments of the retina and retinal pigment epithelium may be seen clinically (Fig. 2-13A).
- Fluorescein angiography is usually not an effective imaging technique, because the fluorescence of the choriocapillaris often masks the vascular lesions (Fig. 2-13B, C).
- Indocyanine green angiography, which better images the choroid, often provides the best visualization of the active lesions. OCT is useful to follow macular involvement.

PROGNOSIS AND MANAGEMENT

- The serosanguineous lesions may resolve spontaneously without progressing to fibrous proliferation. The vascular lesions may involute during periods of disease inactivity, making diagnosis difficult. In contrast, the vascular lesions may continue to grow and repeatedly bleed. These lesions may then develop fibrovascular scarring. Patients may suffer severe visual loss. Treatment for systemic hypertension, if associated with PCV, may be important in limiting the severity of the disease.

● Laser photocoagulation can be considered, especially for serosanguineous complications under the fovea. Treatment to the active polypoidal CNV or to the aneurysmal changes outside the fovea often leads to regression of the entire lesion. This is unlike the experience with CNV due to age-related macular degeneration, in which the entire lesion must be treated to prevent further hemorrhagic complications.

● Intravitreal anti-VEGF agents have limited effectiveness in PCV, although a trial is often utilized with macular involvement. Anti-VEGF therapy may have more effect as adjunctive therapy to other modalities. Ocular photodynamic therapy may be considered for subfoveal lesions.

FIGURE 2-13. Polypoidal choroidal vasculopathy (PCV). A. Areas of serosanguineous retinal detachment in the macula (*arrows*).

(*continued*)

FIGURE 2-13. (*Continued*) **Polypoidal choroidal vasculopathy (PCV). B.** Venous filling phase fluorescein angiogram showing network of branching choroidal vessels (*arrows*). **C.** Late-phase fluorescein angiogram showing leakage of dye in the choroid and terminal aneurysmal dilations.

DEGENERATIVE MYOPIA

Degenerative myopia describes a retinal degenerative condition that consists of thinning of the retinal pigment epithelium and choroid, retinal pigment epithelial atrophy, CNV, and subretinal hemorrhage in patients with progressive elongation of the eye from myopia usually greater than 6 diopters.

EPIDEMIOLOGY AND ETIOLOGY

- The prevalence of degenerative myopia varies among different races and ethnic groups.
- Degenerative myopia is more prevalent in women than in men.

HISTORY

- Patients with degenerative myopia may slowly lose central vision due to progressive atrophy of the macular region. More abrupt vision loss may occur from macular subretinal hemorrhage or CNV.
- Spontaneous improvement in vision may occur if subretinal hemorrhage not associated with CNV resorbs.

IMPORTANT CLINICAL SIGNS

- The clinical findings of degenerative myopia are thought to be due to progressive elongation of the globe. The hallmark finding is the so-called myopic crescent of retinal pigment epithelial atrophy adjacent to the optic nerve (Fig. 2-14A). This atrophic area is usually at the temporal aspect of the disc. However, the atrophy may be located anywhere around the circumference of the disc and may extend through the central macula.

The disc itself may be vertically elongated or tilted, or both (Fig. 2-14B).

- Central macular abnormalities may lead to visual loss. Gyrate areas of atrophy in the posterior pole may involve the foveal region. Lacquer cracks, which are spontaneous linear breaks in Bruch's membrane, may be located in the fovea (see Fig. 2-14B). Lacquer cracks are present in 4% of highly myopic eyes. Spontaneous subretinal hemorrhage without CNV may arise from lacquer cracks (Fig. 2-14C). Fuchs' spots are round areas of subretinal hyperpigmentation, occasionally with surrounding atrophy, that are thought to represent areas of previous subretinal hemorrhage or CNV. Fuchs' spots are seen in 10% of highly myopic eyes after the age of 30.

ASSOCIATED CLINICAL SIGNS

- CNV develops in 5% to 10% of eyes with an axial length greater than 26.5 mm (Fig. 2-14D). CNV is often seen in association with lacquer cracks. Posterior pole staphyloma, an excavation in the posterior pole associated with chorioretinal atrophy, may be present (Fig. 2-14E).
- Diffuse pigmentary alteration and patchy or diffuse areas of chorioretinal degeneration may be present in the retinal periphery (Fig. 2-14F, G). PVD is more common and occurs at an earlier age in patients with degenerative myopia. Although lattice degeneration is not more common in degenerative myopia, patients are at an increased risk of retinal tear and retinal detachment.

DIFFERENTIAL DIAGNOSIS

- Tilted disc syndrome
- Optic disc coloboma

- Presumed ocular histoplasmosis
- Age-related macular degeneration
- Gyrate atrophy

DIAGNOSTIC EVALUATION

- History, refractive error, and axial length measurement in association with the myriad findings on ophthalmoscopy all aid in the diagnosis of degenerative myopia.
- Fluorescein angiography and OCT are helpful to assess for CNV.

PROGNOSIS AND MANAGEMENT

- There are no proven therapies to prevent the progression of myopia and its

degenerative effects upon the retina. Scleral reinforcement and resection techniques have been reported to limit the elongation of the globe, but stabilization or improvement in vision has not been decisively demonstrated.

- Anti-VEGF therapy is effective in treating eyes with myopic CNV. Laser photocoagulation is a second line therapy, and should be considered carefully as the CNV often remains small without treatment. Furthermore, spreading of the atrophic photocoagulation lesion may lead to further visual loss.
- Ocular photodynamic therapy with verteporfin for subfoveal CNV may be useful.
- CNV lesions in degenerative myopia, in distinction from those in age-related macular degeneration, may remain stable without significant visual loss when no treatment is applied.

FIGURE 2-14. **Degenerative myopia. A.** Temporal myopic crescent. Note "thinning" of retinal pigment epithelium (inset reveals true borders of optic nerve).

(continued)

FIGURE 2-14. (*Continued*) **Degenerative myopia. B.** Prominent tilted disc with temporal crescent and lacquer crack above fovea (*arrow*). **C.** Spontaneous subretinal (foveal) hemorrhage from lacquer crack without choroidal neovascularization (CNV).

(*continued*)

FIGURE 2-14. (*Continued*) **Degenerative myopia. D.** Subfoveal CNV (*arrow*) with pigmentation and shallow subretinal fluid. **E.** A posterior staphyloma is present around the optic nerve.

(*continued*)

FIGURE 2-14. (*Continued*) **Degenerative myopia. F.** Extensive chorioretinal atrophy in posterior pole and periphery in the right eye. **G.** Extensive chorioretinal atrophy in posterior pole and periphery in the left eye.

ANGIOID STREAKS

Angioid streaks are red or brown irregular lines that radiate from the optic nerve head. They represent breaks in thickened and calcified Bruch's membrane.

EPIDEMIOLOGY AND ETIOLOGY

● Angioid streaks are idiopathic 50% of the time but are also seen in association with certain systemic diseases. The systemic disease most commonly associated with angioid streaks is pseudoxanthoma elasticum, or Grönblad–Strandberg syndrome. Other systemic conditions associated with angioid streaks are Paget's disease of bone, sickle cell anemia, and Ehlers–Danlos syndrome.

HISTORY

● Patients are asymptomatic unless they develop CNV in association with their angioid streaks. When CNV develops, patients complain of decreased and distorted central vision.

IMPORTANT CLINICAL SIGNS

● Angioid streaks may appear as light red-orange to dark red-brown. The streaks may form a concentric ring around the optic nerve (Fig. 2-15). They may extend through the macula and into the periphery. They may be thin or four times the width of retinal vessels. They are usually bilateral. Over time the streaks may become more atrophic.

ASSOCIATED CLINICAL SIGNS

● CNV can be associated with angioid streaks (Fig. 2-16) and is the leading cause of vision loss due to rupture of the CNV, subretinal hemorrhage, and scarring (Fig. 2-17).

● Patients with pseudoxanthoma elasticum may have an additional fundus finding. There may be a fine stippled appearance to the fundus referred to as *peau d'orange* (like skin of an orange) most commonly seen in the temporal midperiphery (Fig. 2-18).

   ■ Patients with this disease have abnormal dermal elastic tissue. They have loose skin folds in the neck and on the flexor aspects of joints. They may suffer cardiovascular disease from abnormal elastic tissue in blood vessel walls. They may develop gastrointestinal bleeding.

● Patients with Paget's disease (osteitis deformans) have abnormal bone destruction and formation. They typically suffer from headache, enlarged skull, enlarged digits, bone fractures, and cardiovascular complications. Approximately 10% of patients with Paget's disease develop angioid streaks late in the course of their disease. These patients may also suffer visual loss from optic nerve compression by enlarging bone.

● Angioid streaks develop in 1% to 2% of patients with sickle cell hemoglobinopathy. Patients with Ehlers–Danlos syndrome have hyperelasticity of the skin and hyperflexibility of the joints due to abnormal collagen organization.

DIFFERENTIAL DIAGNOSIS

● Traumatic choroidal rupture

DIAGNOSTIC EVALUATION

● In the early phase of fluorescein angiography angioid streaks appear as hyperfluorescent lines due to atrophy of the overlying retinal pigment epithelium. As in any condition associated with disruption of Bruch's membrane, CNV may occur. Typical findings of early hyperfluorescence of CNV with leakage may be seen on fluorescein angiography.

PROGNOSIS AND MANAGEMENT

- When patients have angioid streaks, they remain at risk for CNV. There are no measures available to prevent the development of CNV. If patients develop extrafoveal or juxtafoveal CNV, intravitreal anti-VEGF and/or standard laser photocoagulation can be considered. Ocular photodynamic therapy may become useful for patients with subfoveal CNV in association with angioid streaks that is resistant to anti-VEGF therapy.

- Patients with angioid streaks should be particularly cautious regarding ocular trauma (Fig. 2-19). Safety glasses should be worn because these patients are more susceptible to choroidal rupture and hemorrhage from direct blows to the eye. Patients with angioid streaks should have a general medical evaluation to assess for systemic associations, especially because some of the manifestations, such as cardiovascular disease and gastrointestinal bleeding, are potentially life threatening.

FIGURE 2-15. **Angioid streaks, orange streaks.** Orange lines around the optic nerve with extensions throughout the posterior pole.

FIGURE 2-16. Angioid streaks. A. Subretinal hemorrhage and retinal elevation adjacent to angioid streak is highly suggestive of choroidal neovascularization. **B.** Fluorescein angiogram confirms choroidal neovascularization.

FIGURE 2-17. Angioid streaks, CNV. Severe macular scarring after rupture of CNV and hemorrhage (note peau d'orange appearance temporally).

FIGURE 2-18. Angioid streaks. A. Pigmented streaks with subretinal hemorrhage.

(*continued*)

FIGURE 2-18. (*Continued*) **Angioid streaks. B.** Peau d'orange appearance in the temporal periphery.

FIGURE 2-19. **Angioid streaks, traumatic subretinal hemorrhage.** Patient with bilateral angioid streaks (**A,** right eye; **B,** left eye) was punched in the left eye and suffered extensive subretinal hemorrhage. The subretinal hemorrhage eventually resolved, but left severe scarring (**C**) and visual loss.

(*continued*)

FIGURE 2-19. (*Continued*)

CENTRAL SEROUS RETINOPATHY

CSR is a disease in which a circumscribed serous detachment of the neurosensory retina develops, usually confined to the posterior pole. There may be an associated serous detachment of the retinal pigment epithelium. CSR is usually an idiopathic condition but may be seen in the setting of corticosteroid use.

EPIDEMIOLOGY AND ETIOLOGY

● CSR usually occurs in healthy young to middle-aged men, although women may also be affected. The exact etiology of CSR is unknown. A diffuse abnormality of the retinal pigment epithelium and choroid is likely because fluid resorption is impaired. Recent evidence indicates a possible link to active gastrointestinal *Helicobacter pylori* infection, although this association needs to be substantiated.

● CSR is reportedly more common in patients with a so-called type A personality. Patients being treated with corticosteroids can have particularly severe CSR.

HISTORY

● Patients may be asymptomatic unless the central macula is involved. Symptomatic patients experience sudden onset of decreased central vision with metamorphopsia. There may be macropsia or micropsia. Color vision is often affected, and patients may notice a relative scotoma.

IMPORTANT CLINICAL SIGNS

● On fundus examination patients will have an elevation in the macula due to serous detachment (Fig. 2-20). Patients with chronic or recurrent episodes may have patches of retinal pigment epithelial atrophy.

ASSOCIATED CLINICAL SIGNS

● There may be yellow spots; subretinal precipitates of fibrin deep to the detached retina (Fig. 2-21).

● Often patients will have pigment epithelial clumping from prior episodes in either the involved or the fellow eye, or both (Fig. 2-22).

● Occasionally patients will have an associated serous detachment of the retinal pigment epithelium (Fig. 2-23).

● Rarely patients will have diffuse detachment of the posterior pole with gravity-dependent pooling of fluid inferiorly (Fig. 2-24). This may lead to "gutters" of retinal pigment epithelial alterations created by subretinal fluid that gravitates inferiorly.

DIFFERENTIAL DIAGNOSIS

● CNV, especially in older patients

● Optic nerve pit with neurosensory macular retinal detachment

● Posterior scleritis

● Harada's disease

● Rhegmatogenous retinal detachment

● Circumscribed choroidal hemangioma

● Amelanotic choroidal melanoma

DIAGNOSTIC EVALUATION

● A variety of fluorescein angiographic alterations may be seen in CSR. An expanding dot of hyperfluorescence is the most common alteration (Fig. 2-25). As the angiogram progresses, there is a spot of increasing hyper-fluorescence at the level of the retinal pigment epithelium. In the late phase of the study, there is pooling of dye in the neurosensory detachment.

- Another less common pattern of hyperfluorescence is a "smokestack" appearance in which dye spreads vertically from the retinal pigment epithelium (Fig. 2-26A-D). Occasionally, multiple leakage spots will be seen.

PROGNOSIS AND MANAGEMENT

- Implicated corticosteroids should be immediately discontinued. Most patients undergo spontaneous resolution in 1 to 3 months. However, there may be mild residual symptoms, including decreased central acuity,

reduced contrast sensitivity, decreased color vision, and metamorphopsia. Rarely, patients have severe visual loss. Recurrences happen in 20% to 40% of patients.

- If patients have persistent decreased vision with persistent fluid beyond 3 to 4 months, photocoagulation can be offered to the leak spot seen on fluorescein angiography (Fig. 2-26E).

- Alternatively, there has been recent success with the use of intravitreal anti-VEGF agents for the treatment of persistent CSR. For unresponsive subfoveal lesions, photodynamic therapy can be considered. Patients with occupational needs for improved vision or return of stereoacuity can be considered for earlier treatment. Careful follow-up after laser photocoagulation is necessary because patients may develop CNV at the treatment site.

FIGURE 2-20. **Central serous retinopathy, serous macular detachment.** Serous retinal detachment in the macula.

FIGURE 2-21. Central serous retinopathy, fibrin formation. Subretinal fibrin precipitation in serous detachment of the macula (*arrow*).

FIGURE 2-22. Central serous retinopathy, retinal pigment epithelial alterations. Retinal pigment epithelial clumping in the macula following resolution of serous detachment (inset).

FIGURE 2-23. **Central serous retinopathy. A.** Earlier phase of disease in same patient as in Fig. 2-22. Note serous detachment of the retinal pigment epithelial superotemporal to the optic nerve and fibrin accumulation in the serous detachment of the macula. **B.** Fluorescein angiogram confirms serous detachment of retinal pigment epithelium adjacent to optic nerve.

FIGURE 2-24. Central serous retinopathy. A and **B.** Patient with recurrent CSR (note small serous detachment of macula) who had prior episode(s) of serous detachment that led to gravity-dependent pooling of fluid inferiorly as evidenced by retinal pigment epithelial alterations extending into the inferior periphery.

(*continued*)

FIGURE 2-24. (*Continued*) **Central serous retinopathy. C** and **D.** Fluorescein angiogram showing hyperfluorescence extending from the macula to the inferior periphery due to retinal pigment epithelial alterations from fluid pooling.

FIGURE 2-25. **Central serous retinopathy. A.** Large serous detachment of the macula with fibrin under retina. **B, C** and **D.** Progressive enlargement of spot of hyperfluorescence on fluorescein angiography (*arrow*).

(*continued*)

FIGURE 2-25. (*Continued*)

FIGURE 2-26. Central serous retinopathy, "smokestack" leakage. A. Small serous detachment of the macula with retinal pigment epithelial alterations. **B** and **C.** "Smokestack" appearance of dye leakage on fluorescein angiography.

(*continued*)

FIGURE 2-26. (*Continued*) **Central serous retinopathy, "smokestack" leakage. D.** Fluorescein angiogram showing multiple leakage spots of both the expanding dot and "smokestack" type of leakage.

(*continued*)

FIGURE 2-26. (*Continued*) **Central serous retinopathy, post–laser treatment. E.** Ten weeks after laser photocoagulation. There is complete resolution of subretinal fluid but residual retinal pigment epithelial alterations. Vision improved from 6/30 to 6/9.

CHOROIDAL FOLDS

Folding or wrinkling of the inner choroid, Bruch's membrane, retinal pigment epithelium, and inner retina is known as choroidal or chorioretinal folds.

EPIDEMIOLOGY AND ETIOLOGY

- Choroidal folds are usually idiopathic, but they can be seen in association with other ocular abnormalities, including:
  - Hyperopia
  - Orbital tumors
  - Posterior scleritis
  - Scleral buckling surgery
  - Choroidal tumors
  - Hypotony
  - CNV
  - Chorioretinal scarring
- They may be unilateral or bilateral.

HISTORY

- Patients with long-standing choroidal folds are usually entirely asymptomatic. Those with acute onset of folds are usually symptomatic, with decreased vision and metamorphopsia.

IMPORTANT CLINICAL SIGNS

- Alternating light and dark streaks are seen in the posterior pole in patients with choroidal folds (Fig. 2-27A). The folds may be horizontal, vertical, or oblique in orientation (Fig. 2-27B).

ASSOCIATED CLINICAL SIGNS

- There may be no associated findings if the folds are idiopathic or associated with hyperopia. If there is another ocular condition, then there may be additional signs related to the cause of the folds, such as proptosis in association with an orbital tumor.

DIFFERENTIAL DIAGNOSIS

- Retinal folds (e.g., from macular epiretinal membrane or retinal detachment)

DIAGNOSTIC EVALUATION

- On fluorescein angiography, alternating hyperfluorescent and hypofluorescent bands are seen. The crests of the folds are hyperfluorescent, and the troughs hypofluorescent (Fig. 2-27C).

FIGURE 2-27. Choroidal folds. A. Alternating light and dark streaks through the macula. **B.** Obliquely oriented alternating light and dark streaks above the macula.

(continued)

FIGURE 2-27. (*Continued*) **Choroidal folds. C.** Fluorescein angiogram showing alternating hyperfluorescent and hypofluorescent bands.

HYPOTONY MACULOPATHY

- Hypotony maculopathy is a condition in which chorioretinal folds develop in the posterior pole of patients with chronically low intraocular pressure.

EPIDEMIOLOGY AND ETIOLOGY

- Patients with chronically low intraocular pressure from a wound leak, cyclodialysis cleft, or excessive filtering after glaucoma surgery may develop secondary retinal changes.

HISTORY

- Patients will experience loss of central vision from the chorioretinal folds.

IMPORTANT CLINICAL SIGNS

- Broad chorioretinal folds radiate out temporally from the optic nerve in a branching fashion (**Fig. 2-28**). Nasally the folds are usually arranged concentric to the optic nerve or have an irregular arrangement.
- The macular retina may be thrown into radiating folds around the fovea distinct from the choroidal folds.
- The peripapillary choroid is often swollen, mimicking optic disc edema.

ASSOCIATED CLINICAL SIGNS

- The intraocular pressure will be low, usually less than 5 mm Hg. There may be anterior segment signs consistent with surgery or trauma.

DIFFERENTIAL DIAGNOSIS

- Chorioretinal folds from other causes:
  - Idiopathic
  - Hyperopia
  - Orbital tumors
  - Posterior scleritis
  - Scleral buckling surgery
  - Choroidal tumors
  - Hypotony
  - CNV
  - Chorioretinal scarring

DIAGNOSTIC EVALUATION

- Fluorescein angiography will demonstrate alternating hypofluorescent and hyperfluorescent lines corresponding to the folds. Optic disc hyperfluorescence and macular leakage may be observed.
- OCT is helpful in diagnosing patients with reduced vision and an otherwise normal exam. OCT may reveal the retinal folds or macular edema.

PROGNOSIS AND MANAGEMENT

- Surgical correction of the underlying cause of hypotony maculopathy will usually result in resolution of the folds and visual improvement. Long-standing folds may resolve with treatment, but there may be residual linear retinal pigment epithelial alterations from the chronic folding of the retinal pigment epithelium.

FIGURE 2-28. Hypotony maculopathy. Horizontal and oblique macular folds in a patient with hypotony maculopathy after glaucoma surgery.

Diabetic Retinopathy

James F. Vander

DIABETIC RETINOPATHY

Diabetic retinopathy encompasses a broad range of fundus manifestations of diabetes mellitus. This is a clinical term that includes exudative, hemorrhagic, ischemic, proliferative, and tractional manifestations of this retinal vascular disease. It can be arbitrarily divided into a nonproliferative and a proliferative form.

EPIDEMIOLOGY AND ETIOLOGY

- Diabetic retinopathy is the leading cause of blindness in the United States and Western Europe among adults less than age 55 years. It affects both genders and all races, although African Americans are more frequently and more severely affected than Caucasians.
- The best predictor of diabetic retinopathy is the duration of disease. For type 1 diabetic patients there is no risk of retinopathy for roughly 5 years after initial diagnosis. Some retinopathy is present in up to 50% of patients 10 years after diagnosis. After 15 years, 95% of patients show some retinopathy. Proliferative retinopathy is very uncommon with less than 10 years' duration of disease. Forty percent of patients have proliferative disease by 25 years.
- The trend for type 2 diabetic patients is very similar. Many patients will have asymptomatic, occult diabetes for many years prior to diagnosis, however, and therefore may present with retinopathy even at the time of diagnosis of diabetes mellitus.
- Age is another important risk factor in the prevalence of diabetic retinopathy. Diabetic retinopathy is very rare prior to puberty. Its prevalence increases dramatically after puberty, however, and over 50% of patients will develop retinopathy by their early twenties.

PATHOPHYSIOLOGY

- Hyperglycemia is a key factor in the development of diabetic retinopathy. The mechanism of retinopathy development may be related to:
  - Relative hypercoagulability
  - Red blood cell abnormalities

- Excessive glycosylation of proteins
- Enzymatic conversion of excessive glucose by aldose reductase
- Histopathologically, thickening of retinal capillary basement membranes and loss of pericytes have been shown consistently.

HISTORY

- Patients are often asymptomatic but may have blurry vision or floaters. More extensive visual loss occurs with large vitreous hemorrhages or retinal detachment.

NONPROLIFERATIVE DIABETIC RETINOPATHY

IMPORTANT CLINICAL SIGNS

- *Nonproliferative Diabetic retinopathy* (NPDR) is the preferred term for this less severe manifestation of diabetic retinopathy. It may be arbitrarily subdivided into mild, moderate, and severe categories.

Mild Nonproliferative Diabetic Retinopathy

- Earliest fundus manifestations of diabetic retinopathy. Features reflect retinal capillary hyperpermeability. May be manifested as:
  - Intraretinal hemorrhage—dot hemorrhages are small mid-level retinal hemorrhages (Fig. 3-1).
  - Blot hemorrhages—larger, with fuzzier borders.
  - Flame-shaped hemorrhages—superficial in the nerve fiber layer.
  - Microaneurysms—saccular enlargement of retinal capillaries.
  - Lipoprotein exudation—also known as hard yellow exudate (HYE; Figs. 3-2 and 3-3).

- Macular edema—the most common reason for legal blindness resulting from diabetic retinopathy. It is best appreciated as macular thickening by the use of a high magnification slit-lamp examination using a hand held or contact lens providing a good stereoscopic view (Fig. 3-4).

Moderate Nonproliferative Diabetic Retinopathy

- This degree of retinopathy is characterized by increased number and size of intraretinal hemorrhaging with greater evidence for exudation as manifested by more HYE (Fig. 3-5) and macular edema than is present in mild nonproliferative retinopathy. (Standardized photographs exist to establish the transition points between the various stages of nonproliferative retinopathy, but it should be remembered that this classification reflects a continuum of disease severity.) In moderate nonproliferative retinopathy one also begins to see evidence of capillary occlusive disease. This is reflected by the development of:
  - Cotton-wool spots (Fig. 3-6)
  - Venous dilation and beading (Fig. 3-7)
  - Intraretinal microvascular abnormality (IRMA)—flat, intraretinal, irregular blood vessel. (It is sometimes difficult to distinguish between IRMA and neovascularization of the retina. Fluorescein angiography can be helpful in making this distinction; Fig. 3-8B.)

- Vision loss in moderate NPDR may be the result of macular edema or, less frequently, loss of some of the normal perifoveolar capillary bed. Frequently, both problems may be present.

Severe Nonproliferative Retinopathy

- In severe NPDR there is worsening of the exudative aspect of diabetic retinopathy and, especially, evidence for capillary occlusive changes. More extensive intraretinal hemorrhaging, venous beading, IRMA, as well

TABLE 3-1. 4-2-1 Rule

The presence of:

   Severe retinal hemorrhages in **4** quadrants

   or

   Venous beading in **2** quadrants

   or

   IRMA in **1** quadrant

Indicates a 50% risk of developing proliferative retinopathy within 1 year

as edema and exudate are the features that define severe nonproliferative retinopathy (**Figs. 3-8 to 3-10**). The presence of certain fundus features predicts the progression toward proliferative retinopathy (**Table 3-1**).

ASSOCIATED CLINICAL SIGNS

• Cornea—decrease of corneal sensitivity; increased risk abrasion

• Cataract—typically nuclear and cortical cataract formation is chronic and progressive; acute cortical cataract formation with profound elevations in blood glucose

• Glaucoma—greater incidence of primary open-angle glaucoma

• Cranial nerve palsy—isolated palsy, most often sixth

DIFFERENTIAL DIAGNOSIS

• Other causes of retinal capillary leakage and occlusion include:

  ▪ Hypertensive retinopathy

  ▪ Retinal vein occlusion (branch or central) (**Fig. 3-11**)

  ▪ Hemoglobinopathies

  ▪ Anemia or leukemia

  ▪ Ocular ischemic syndrome

  ▪ Radiation retinopathy (**Fig. 3-12**)

  ▪ Idiopathic juxtafoveal telangiectasis

  ▪ Coats' disease

  ▪ Vasculitis (e.g., sarcoidosis, lupus)

DIAGNOSTIC EVALUATION

• The most important aspect of the evaluation of NPDR is a magnified, stereoscopic, slit-lamp biomicroscopic examination of the posterior pole and midperipheral retina using a handheld indirect lens or contact lens. A critical determination is the presence or absence of clinically significant macular edema (CSME; **Table 3-2**).

• Fluorescein angiography is a valuable ancillary test in evaluation of NPDR. Indications include:

  ▪ Determination of location of focal and diffuse leakage to guide treatment (**Fig. 3-13**)

  ▪ Rule out loss of perifoveal capillaries

  ▪ Mechanism for unexplained vision loss

  ▪ Risk factor for vision loss after focal laser

  ▪ Rule out vasculitis or other diagnostic possibilities

TABLE 3-2. Clinically Significant Macular Edema (CSME)

Retinal thickening within 500 μm center of fovea

   or

Exudate within 500 μm center of fovea with adjacent thickening

   or

Thickening of at least one disc area any part within one disc diameter of center of fovea

Note: CSME is a diagnosis based on stereoscopic macular viewing independent of visual acuity or fluorescein angiography.

- Optical coherence tomography (OCT) is another ancillary test that is important in managing diabetic macular edema. OCT provides a noncontrast, photographic method for determining the presence of fluid within and under the retina, quantifying the extent of that fluid and monitor the response to therapy (Fig. 3-14).

PROGNOSIS AND MANAGEMENT

- NPDR tends to progress gradually over months to years. The risk of vision loss increases with increasing severity of retinopathy. Treatment of systemic disease reduces but does not eliminate the risk of progression and vision loss (Table 3-3). Newer medications under development may actually reverse retinopathy.
- Ocular treatment consists of macular laser photocoagulation for macular edema (Fig. 3-15). Early treatment diabetic retinopathy study (ETDRS) guidelines are widely applied (Table 3-4). The utility and timing of retreatment, the role of early treatment before ETDRS threshold is reached, and the application of alternative treatment strategies are less uniformly accepted.
- The ETDRS addressed three questions:
  1. What is the role of aspirin in diabetic retinopathy? *Answer:* It neither improves nor worsens retinopathy.

TABLE 3-3. Diabetes Control and Complications Trial (DCCT)

DCCT showed that tightened blood glucose control reduces:

Development of retinopathy by 76%

Progression of retinopathy by 80%

Risk of nephropathy by about 60%

Risk of neuropathy by about 60%

TABLE 3-4. Early Treatment Diabetic Retinopathy Study (ETDRS) Facts

ETDRS treatment of macular edema:

Generally stabilizes visual acuity but often does not improve it

Consists of directly treating focal areas of leakage and placing a grid in areas of diffuse capillary leakage; determination of treatment placement is generally guided by the use of a fluorescein angiogram

Should be avoided in the presence of significant loss of perifoveal capillaries

May take months to show resolution of thickening and longer for exudates

2. What is the role of initiating early laser (as compared to DRS high-risk criteria; Table 3-5) in the management of severe nonproliferative and early proliferative retinopathy? *Answer:* Inconclusive. No strong benefit to early scatter panretinal photocoagulation (PRP) was found. Certain clinical circumstances (e.g., poor compliance with follow-up examinations, rapid progression in fellow eye) may justify early initiation of PRP.

3. What is the role of laser (PRP or focal macular laser, or both) in the management of macular edema? *Answer:* There is no role for PRP in treatment of macular edema. Macular laser is of benefit, reducing the risk of moderate visual loss by 50%. Patients with CSME should be treated.

TABLE 3-5. Diabetic Retinopathy Clinical Research (DRCR)

- Macular laser photocoagulation is superior to repeated intravitreal injection of triamcinolone acetonide for primary treatment of macular edema in general.
- Ranibizumab injections are as good (? better) as laser for treatment of CSME at 1 year

• More recently, the use of intravitreal injection of pharmacologic agents has provided an alternative method for treating macular edema. The diabetic retinopathy clinical research (DRCR) studies have assessed the utility of some of these agents (**Table 3-5**). Intravitreal triamcinolone acetonide causes a rapid reduction of macular edema and subretinal fluid in most cases. The effect is generally temporary and side effects include cataract progression and elevation of intraocular pressure, sometimes markedly. DRCR results suggest that steroid injection is not as effective as macular laser for primary treatment of edema.

• More recently, injection of anti-VEGF agents bevacizumab and ranibizumab have shown a strong positive therapeutic effect with repeated injections (**Fig. 3-16**). The DRCR preliminary results suggest that ranibizumab may be superior to focal laser as primary treatment, at least for 12 months. These indications are evolving.

FIGURE 3-1. Minimal nonproliferative diabetic retinopathy (NPDR).

FIGURE 3-2. NPDR with retinal hemorrhages and hard yellow exudates (HYEs).

FIGURE 3-3. Subtle HYE near fovea in NPDR.

FIGURE 3-4. **A.** Retinal hemorrhages, HYE, and edema in NPDR. **B.** Venous phase intravenous fluorescein angiogram (IVFA) showing numerous microaneurysms seen as pinpoint dots of hyperfluorescence.

(*continued*)

FIGURE 3-4. (*Continued*) **C.** Leakage from microaneurysms with obscuration of hyperfluorescent dots. **D.** Later phase showing more extensive leakage.

FIGURE 3-5. Macular edema and HYE with blunting of foveal reflex.

FIGURE 3-6. Cotton-wool spots as well as hemorrhage and HYE.

FIGURE 3-7. Venous beading (*arrow*) indicating more severe NPDR.

FIGURE 3-8. **A.** Severe NPDR.

(*continued*)

FIGURE 3-8. (*Continued*) **B.** IVFA shows numerous microaneurysms and patches of capillary nonperfusion (arrowhead). Note abnormal vessels (intraretinal microvascular abnormality, IRMA) along superotemporal arcade (*arrowhead*). **C.** High-powered view of IRMA seen in **B.** Absence of leakage distinguishes IRMA from neovascularization.

FIGURE 3-9. Sausaging of retinal venules (*arrow*) seen in severe NPDR.

FIGURE 3-10. Venous loop.

FIGURE 3-11. Hemorrhages and cotton-wool spots in branch retinal vein obstruction. Note the segmental distribution of the fundus abnormalities.

FIGURE 3-12. Numerous cotton-wool spots with a few hemorrhages in a nondiabetic patient with a history of prior radiation for treatment of a brain tumor.

FIGURE 3-13. A. Retinal hemorrhages with mild macular edema. **B.** Enlargement of the foveal avascular zone with microaneurysms near the center of the macula (inset).

(continued)

FIGURE 3-13. (*Continued*) **C.** Late leakage from the microaneurysms.

FIGURE 3-14. OCT shows cystic edema in central macula.

FIGURE 3-15. A. Macular edema and HYE in NPDR. **B.** Several months after laser treatment, resolution of edema and HYE is seen.

FIGURE 3-16. **A.** OCT shows cystic macular edema. **B.** One week after intravitreal bevacizumab there is marked reduction in macular thickening.

PROLIFERATIVE DIABETIC RETINOPATHY

Proliferative diabetic retinopathy (PDR) represents the most severe manifestation of diabetes in the eye. It is the result of the loss of normal retinal perfusion and the subsequent development of neovascular proliferative tissue in the fundus. The development of this neovascular tissue reflects an alteration in the balance between angiogenesis inhibitors and stimulators in the retina and vitreous. Multiple local chemical mediators (cytokines) are believed to be at work.

IMPORTANT CLINICAL SIGNS

- **Neovascularization of the disc (NVD):** Neovascularization that develops on the surface of the optic nerve or within one disc diameter of the optic nerve is defined as NVD (**Figs. 3-17 to 3-19;** see also **Fig. 3-21**). Shunt vessels that may develop on the optic disc (e.g., after a retinal venous obstruction) may be easily confused with NVD. Neovascularization of the disc typically has a lacy irregular appearance and may be elevated above the optic nerve surface. True NVD should be distinguished from the hyperemic disc swelling of diabetic papillopathy.

- **Neovascularization elsewhere (NVE):** This term refers to retinal neovascularization anywhere in the fundus that is not NVD (**Figs. 3-20 and 3-21**). Neovascularization elsewhere in PDR tends to occur in the posterior pole or midperiphery, although extreme peripheral NVE can also develop. Neovascularization elsewhere tends to form at the junction between perfused and nonperfused retina, and this can be readily appreciated with fluorescein angiography.

- **Neovascularization of the iris (NVI):** Development of NVI is an ominous sign

(**Fig. 3-22**). Involvement of the anterior chamber angle can produce neovascular glaucoma (NVG), leading to a blind, painful eye.

- **Vitreous hemorrhage:** Bleeding from NVD or NVE may occur and produce preretinal or vitreous hemorrhage. Vitreous hemorrhage is more likely when NVD and NVE are more extensive. Hemorrhages are usually spontaneous and produce a sudden development of floaters. Preretinal hemorrhage reflects sequestration of blood between the inner retinal surface and an intact posterior hyaloid face (**Fig. 3-23**). Therefore, this will generally occur in younger patients. This may produce a dense, well-circumscribed scotoma (**Figs. 3-24 and 3-25**). Often preretinal hemorrhage will subsequently break apart and produce more diffuse floaters characteristic of vitreous hemorrhage (**Figs. 3-26 and 3-27**). Vitreous hemorrhage is often recurrent and can produce profound visual loss.

MANAGEMENT

- The treatment of proliferative retinopathy is guided by the diabetic retinopathy study (DRS; **Tables 3-6 and 3-7**). Laser PRP as

TABLE 3-6. Diabetic Retinopathy Study (DRS)

DRS showed:

Risk features for severe visual loss (defined as visual acuity of 5/200 or worse) are:

NVD > ⅓ to ¼ of disc area

Any NVD with associated VH

NVE with associated VH

These features are known as **high-risk characteristics** (HRC). Patients with HRC treated with PRP have a 50% reduction in risk of severe visual loss.

NVD, neovascularization of the disc; NVE, neovascularization elsewhere; PRP, panretinal photocoagulation; VH, vitreous hemorrhage.

TABLE 3-7. Panretinal Photocoagulation (PRP) Facts

PRP:

Does not improve visual acuity

May cause worsening macular edema, and loss of peripheral vision and night vision

Indications for supplementation are uncertain

Does not always cause regression of NVD/NVE

Is also indicated in patients with NVI from PDR even in the absence of NVD/NVE

NVD, neovascularization of the disc; NVE, neovascularization elsewhere; NVI, neovascularization of the iris; PDR, proliferative diabetic retinopathy.

established by the DRS is the treatment of choice (**Figs. 3-28 to 3-30**).

● For eyes with more advanced nonclearing vitreous hemorrhage or fibrovascular scarring, or both, vitrectomy may be indicated. Intravitreal injection of anti-VEGF agents will induce rapid regression of neovascularization. This approach may be utilized as primary treatment, in conjunction with laser photocoagulation or as a pre-operative adjunct to anticipated vitrectomy surgery.

Macular Ischemia

● There is no effective treatment for diabetic macular ischemia. This condition more commonly occurs in eyes with PDR but may be observed in association with nonproliferative disease as well. Irregular enlargement of the foveal avascular zone on fluorescein angiography is observed (**Fig. 3-31**).

Retinal Detachment

● The development of neovascular tissue produces an unusually strong adhesion between the vitreous and retina. With contraction of the vitreous as well as the fibrovascular proliferative tissue, increasing traction on the retina will develop. Sufficient traction may ultimately lead to a retinal detachment. A traction retinal detachment typically has a concave, immobile appearance with retinal striae radiating from the areas of greatest traction. When traction retinal detachment affects the macula, severe visual loss is noted.

● Combined traction and rhegmatogenous retinal detachment may develop if vitreous traction is severe enough to produce a full-thickness retinal break. Combined retinal detachments tend to develop more rapidly than purely tractional retinal detachments. The retina appears more mobile with corrugations and undulations noted with eye movement.

Indications for Vitrectomy in Proliferative Diabetic Retinopathy

● Definite

  ▪ Persistent or recurrent vitreous hemorrhage (see **Figs. 3-25 and 3-26**)

  ▪ Traction macular detachment (**Figs. 3-32 and 3-33**)

  ▪ Combined traction and rhegmatogenous retinal detachment (**Fig. 3-34**)

● Possible

  ▪ Severe proliferation unresponsive to PRP (**Fig. 3-35**)

  ▪ Traction detachment threatening the macula

  ▪ Persistent macular edema with taut posterior hyaloid face

FIGURE 3-17. Neovascularization of the disc (NVD). Moderately severe NVD as defined in the Diabetic Retinopathy Study. (Standard Photo 10A, courtesy of the Diabetic Retinopathy Study Group.)

FIGURE 3-18. Severe elevated NVD.

FIGURE 3-19. A. Proliferative diabetic retinopathy (PDR) with macular edema, HYE, and NVD. **B.** IVFA confirming NVD and enlarged irregular foveal avascular zone.

(*continued*)

FIGURE 3-19. (*Continued*) **C.** Late phase showing marked leakage from NVD and severe macular edema.

FIGURE 3-20. A. Patches of neovascularization elsewhere (NVE). Note the bland appearance of the fundus peripheral to the NVE.

(*continued*)

FIGURE 3-20. (*Continued*) **B.** Macular view on IVFA demonstrates microaneurysms but minimal ischemia. **C.** Hyperfluorescence of the NVE.

(*continued*)

FIGURE 3-20. (*Continued*) **D.** Note the marked capillary nonperfusion peripheral to the NVE.

FIGURE 3-21. **A.** PDR with NVD and NVE (*arrows*).

(*continued*)

FIGURE 3-21. (*Continued*) **B.** IVFA showing hyperfluorescence of NVD and NVE. Note the irregular capillary bed in the central macula (inset). **C.** Marked hyperfluorescence of NVE with peripheral nonperfusion.

(*continued*)

FIGURE 3-21. (*Continued*) **D.** Marked late hyperfluorescence from leaking NVD and NVE with macular edema.

FIGURE 3-22. Neovascularization of the iris in PDR seen through a gonioscopic mirror.

FIGURE 3-23. Mild vitreous hemorrhage in PDR.

FIGURE 3-24. Large preretinal hemorrhage in PDR resulting in a large, dense scotoma.

FIGURE 3-25. Boat-shaped preretinal hemorrhage in PDR.

FIGURE 3-26. More dense vitreous hemorrhage.

FIGURE 3-27. A. Early-phase IVFA showing enlargement of foveal avascular zone in diabetic retinopathy. Note the hyperfluorescent dot inferior to the fovea (*arrow*). **B.** Hyperfluorescence and linear horizontal hypofluorescence develop suddenly during the IVFA as spontaneous preretinal hemorrhage begins to occur from a tiny area of NVE.

(continued)

FIGURE 3-27. (*Continued*) **C.** The area of hyper- and hypofluorescence enlarges as hemorrhage expands during the IVFA. **D.** Red-free photograph showing fresh preretinal hemorrhage. Photo was taken shortly after (**C**).

FIGURE 3-28. Laser photocoagulation scars spaced about one burn width apart in panretinal photocoagulation (PRP).

FIGURE 3-29. PRP scars in PDR. Note sparing of the macula.

FIGURE 3-30. Equator-plus photo after full PRP.

FIGURE 3-31. A. Posterior pole after PRP. The patient had no appreciable macular thickening but vision was reduced to 20/80. **B.** IVFA showing enlarged, irregular foveal avascular zone (inset) identifying ischemia as the mechanism of vision loss.

FIGURE 3-32. A. Traction retinal detachment involving the macula. **B.** Postoperative appearance after vitrectomy, membrane peeling, and PRP.

FIGURE 3-33. **A.** Marked traction on the macula in a patient found to have a full-thickness retinal break as well during vitrectomy. **B.** Postoperative appearance shows the retina to be attached, PRP and a residual vitreous cavity gas bubble (*arrow*) slowly resolving.

FIGURE 3-34. Wide angle photograph showing combined traction and rhegmatogenous retinal disease in PDR. Note the full-thickness retinal hole nasally and adjacent white fibrovascular traction.

FIGURE 3-35. **A.** Preoperative appearance of highly elevated and vascularized NVD. **B.** Two days after intravitreal injection of bevacizumab the NVD looks white and tissue manipulation during vitrectomy is greatly facilitated.

DIABETIC PAPILLOPATHY

Diabetic papillopathy describes optic disc edema, either unilateral or bilateral, in a diabetic patient with evidence for minimal or mild optic nerve dysfunction and no evidence for ocular inflammation or elevated intracranial pressure.

EPIDEMIOLOGY AND ETIOLOGY

- Roughly 70% of patients have type 1 diabetes, and 60% of cases are unilateral.
- Etiology is uncertain, although some suggest a mild nonarteritic anterior ischemic optic neuropathy (AION).

HISTORY

- Patients may have blurry vision or be asymptomatic.
- Rarely there will be transient visual obscuration.
- Neurologic symptoms are absent.

IMPORTANT CLINICAL SIGNS

- Disc swelling occurs with prominent surface vessels and fine hemorrhages on the disc.
- An afferent papillary defect is present but generally not severe.
- Visual loss is often mild with 20/40 or better in 75% of cases.

ASSOCIATED CLINICAL SIGNS

- A crowded optic disc is often present, similar to AION. This does not correlate with the degree of diabetic retinopathy.

DIFFERENTIAL DIAGNOSIS

- Optic disc neovascularization from PDR
- AION
- Optic neuritis
- Optic disc drusen
- Papilledema

DIAGNOSTIC EVALUATION

- In general, no workup is needed in the appropriate clinical setting. If the case is atypical, then imaging such as a magnetic resonance scan is indicated.
- Visual field examination may be useful to document and follow visual loss.
- Fluorescein angiography can distinguish diabetic papillopathy from NVD but is rarely needed. Diabetic papillopathy typically stains without significant leakage on fluorescein angiography whereas NVD shows leakage of dye into the vitreous cavity.

PROGNOSIS AND MANAGEMENT

- No treatment is indicated. Substantial spontaneous recovery occurs, usually over weeks to months, with many patients showing subtle optic atrophy or visual field defects permanently.
- Patients should be monitored to rule out rapid progression to PDR, which occurs in a minority of cases.

Retinal Vascular Disease

Gary C. Brown

COTTON-WOOL SPOTS

Cotton-wool spots describe the retinal change resulting from acute blockage of blood flow within a terminal retinal arteriole.

EPIDEMIOLOGY AND ETIOLOGY

- The prevalence is uncertain. Cotton-wool spots are seen in over 40% of cases of diabetic retinopathy and also with acute systemic arterial hypertension.
- No hereditary pattern is known.

PATHOPHYSIOLOGY

- Embolic
- Hypertensive arteriolar necrosis
- Inflammatory
- See Diagnostic Evaluation below

CLINICAL SIGNS

- Visual acuity: Central visual acuity is usually unaffected, although patients may note the sudden appearance of corresponding blind spots.
- Pupillary changes: An afferent pupillary defect is usually absent.
- Fundus changes: Cotton-wool spots appear in the posterior pole of the fundus (not the peripheral retina) as superficial areas of retinal opacification that characteristically measure less than one quarter disc area in size (Fig. 4-1). When associated with diabetes mellitus, systemic arterial hypertension, and retinal venous obstruction, they are generally seen concomitantly with retinal hemorrhages. Cotton-wool spots usually resolve over 5 to 7 weeks but may remain longer when present in conjunction with diabetic retinopathy.

DIFFERENTIAL DIAGNOSIS

- Inflammatory retinitis may occur from entities such as toxoplasmosis or cytomegalovirus.
- Retinal hemorrhages are typically present with the latter.
- There are also usually vitreous cells present with inflammatory conditions, but not with cotton-wool spots alone.

DIAGNOSTIC EVALUATION

● Intravenous fluorescein angiography is minimally helpful. It reveals areas of relative hypofluorescence corresponding to the cotton-wool spots.

● Systemic workup (similar to that of acute central retinal artery obstruction, unless the obvious causes of diabetic retinopathy, systemic arterial hypertension, and retinal venous obstruction are present):

  ▪ Diabetic retinopathy: Cotton-wool spots are present in 44% of cases.

  ▪ Systemic arterial hypertension: Diastolic blood pressure of 105 to 110 mm Hg or more is usually necessary to induce cotton-wool spot formation in adults.

  ▪ Retinal vein obstruction: Central, branch.

  ▪ Embolic: Carotid and cardiac.

  ▪ Inflammatory: Giant cell arteritis, Wegener's granulomatosis, polyarteritis nodosa, systemic lupus erythematosus, scleroderma, orbital mucormycosis, toxoplasmosis retinitis.

  ▪ Coagulopathies: Sickle cell disease, homocysteinuria, lupus anticoagulant syndrome, protein S deficiency, protein C deficiency, antithrombin III deficiency, and the factor V Leiden mutation.

  ▪ Miscellaneous: Migraine, Lyme disease, hypotension, acquired immunodeficiency syndrome (AIDS), interferon therapy, metastatic carcinoma, intravenous drug abuse (chronic), papilledema, acute pancreatitis, severe anemia, radiation retinopathy, leptospirosis, Purtscher's retinopathy.

PROGNOSIS AND MANAGEMENT

● The visual prognosis for central vision is good unless there are innumerable cotton-wool spots as with entities such as systemic lupus erythematosus, pancreatitis, Purtscher's retinopathy, or intravenous drug abuse. Associated damage from entities that cotton-wool spots accompany (e.g., diabetic retinopathy or retinal venous obstruction) can lead to severe visual loss.

● There is no consistently proven treatment to ameliorate the visual acuity. When known diabetic retinopathy and retinal vein obstruction are excluded as causes, a serious associated systemic disease can be found in 95% of cases. Thus, it is critical to undertake a systemic workup if there is no appreciable underlying cause, even if only one cotton-wool spot is present.

FIGURE 4-1. **Cotton-wool spots.** Multiple cotton-wool spots (inset) in the fundus of a patient with human immunodeficiency virus (HIV) infection.

HYPERTENSIVE RETINOPATHY

Hypertensive retinopathy refers to the retinal vascular changes associated with systemic arterial hypertension. Hypertensive choroidopathy may also accompany the acute phases of hypertensive retinopathy. Blood pressure can vary throughout the day, as can coverage with hypertensive medications. Thus, having a patient measure blood pressure at home three times a day for 3 to 4 days gives the clinician and the patient greater confidence that the blood pressure is either stable or not.

EPIDEMIOLOGY

- Hypertensive retinopathy can be divided into chronic and acute phases. The most commonly used classification is the Keith–Wagener–Barker classification. The grades of hypertensive retinopathy are as follows:

  - Grade 1: Retinal arterial narrowing (Fig. 4-2)
  - Grade 2: Retinal arteriovenous nicking (Fig. 4-3)
  - Grade 3: Retinal hemorrhages, cotton-wool spots, hard exudates (Fig. 4-4)
  - Grade 4: Grade 3 changes plus optic disc swelling (Fig. 4-5)

- Grades 1 and 2 are commonly seen in practice. Grade 3 and 4 changes are much less frequently seen.

PATHOPHYSIOLOGY

- **Grades 1 and 2:** Hyalinization and thickening of the retinal arterial walls is seen, leading to the straightened vessels in grade 1 and the indentation (arteriovenous nicking) of the retinal veins by the arteries in grade 2 hypertensive

retinopathy. Arteriovenous nicking of a retinal vein does not occur at an arteriovenous crossing unless the retinal artery is located anterior to the retinal vein, a phenomenon which occurs in approximately two-thirds of the arteriovenous crossings in the posterior pole.

- **Grade 3:** The systemic diastolic blood pressure in an adult with grade 3 hypertensive retinopathy is typically at least 105 to 110 mm Hg. At this point, the retinal arteries lose their ability to autoregulate the blood flow, and the high pressure is passed distally to the retinal arterioles and capillary bed. This same clinical signs can be seen in children when the systolic blood is in the nineties.

- **Grade 4:** The systemic diastolic blood pressure in an adult with grade 4 hypertensive retinopathy is usually at least 130 to 140 mm Hg. With both grades 3 and 4 hypertensive retinopathy, the increased blood pressure can damage the blood vessel wall, leading to fibrinoid necrosis (the presence of fibrin thrombi within the vascular lumina). A similar process occurs with hypertensive choroidopathy, leading to necrosis of the overlying retinal pigment epithelium (Elschnig spot).

CLINICAL SIGNS

- Grade 1 and 2 changes are chronic, whereas grade 3 and 4 changes indicate acute retinal vascular decompensation.

- Hypertensive choroidopathy (Elschnig spots) may accompany grade 3 and 4 changes. Elschnig spots are round and yellow acutely, eventually changing to pigmented lesions.

DIFFERENTIAL DIAGNOSIS

- Diabetic retinopathy, radiation retinopathy, venous occlusive disease, carotid artery occlusive disease (ocular ischemic syndrome), and collagen vascular diseases can all mimic the changes of hypertensive retinopathy.

DIAGNOSTIC EVALUATION

- Measurement of the systemic blood pressure is critical when the diagnosis is suspected. If the acute changes (grades 3 and 4) are classic and the blood pressure is not elevated at the time of measurement, consideration should be given to the possibility that the blood pressure has been uncontrolled recently or is uncontrolled at other times during the day.

PROGNOSIS AND MANAGEMENT

- Vision is typically unaffected with grades 1 and 2 hypertensive retinopathy and may be mildly decreased with grade 3 retinopathy.

- With grade 4 retinopathy, vision can be markedly decreased due to retinal edema, hard exudates in the central macula (macular star) and/or the presence of a serous retinal detachment.

- The treatment for hypertensive retinopathy is to correct the underlying condition by normalizing the blood pressure. This causes resolution of the fundus abnormalities over a period of weeks to months in eyes with grade 3 and 4 changes, but often does not affect the changes seen with grades 1 and 2 hypertensive retinopathy.

- Laser therapy has not been shown to be of benefit in treating the visual loss associated with grade 3 and 4 hypertensive retinopathy. Correcting the blood pressure after grade 4 retinopathy can lead to visual improvement, although there may be residual, permanent visual loss due to vascular shutdown in hypertensive choroidopathy, hypertensive retinopathy, hypertensive optic neuropathy. Oral nifedipine has been suggested for the treatment of acute grade 4 hypertensive retinopathy.

- Theoretically, intravitreal VEGF-A inhibitor therapy with ranibizumab and/or bevacizumab could stabilize the walls of retinal of vessels with grade 3 or 4 systemic arterial hypertension changes. As of this writing, data on the treatment of hypertensive retinopathy with these interventions are lacking.

- If the blood pressure associated with grade 4 hypertensive retinopathy is untreated, the 18-month mortality rate is 94%.

FIGURE 4-2. **Hypertensive retinopathy, grade 1.** The retinal arteries are markedly narrowed and straightened. Small retinal hemorrhages are present, not due to hypertension but due to background diabetic retinopathy.

FIGURE 4-3. **Hypertensive retinopathy, grade 2.** Prominent arteriovenous nicking (*arrows*) is seen. Small retinal hemorrhages are present, not due to hypertension, but due to diabetic retinopathy.

FIGURE 4-4. **Hypertensive retinopathy, grade 4.** Cotton-wool spots, retinal hemorrhages, a macular star composed of intraretinal lipid exudates, and a serous detachment of the macula are all present. The optic nerve head is swollen, the feature that separates grade 3 and grade 4 hypertensive retinopathy.

FIGURE 4-5. Hypertensive retinopathy, grade 4. A. Retinal hemorrhages are present, the optic disc is swollen, and an exudative retinal detachment (*arrows*) is present inferiorly. Yellow Elschnig spots (asterisk) are present in the macula. **B.** Fluorescein angiogram corresponding to **A.** Profound retinal capillary nonperfusion is present in the macula (macular ischemia), and foci of hyperfluorescence corresponding to the Elschnig spots (asterisk) are also seen in the macula.

(continued)

FIGURE 4-5. (*Continued*) **Hypertensive retinopathy, grade 4. C.** Fluorescein angiogram of the superior fundus of the eye shown in **A.** Numerous foci of hyperfluorescence corresponding to Elschnig spots (asterisk) can be seen.

CILIORETINAL ARTERY OBSTRUCTION (OCCLUSION)

Cilioretinal artery obstruction is the acute blockage of blood flow within a cilioretinal artery.

EPIDEMIOLOGY AND ETIOLOGY

- Cilioretinal artery obstruction typically occurs in patients aged 65 years and older but can be seen at any age.

- It is seen in approximately 1:100,000 outpatient ophthalmology visits.

- The abnormality is unilateral in over 99% of cases. No hereditary pattern is known.

PATHOPHYSIOLOGY

- Embolic
- Hypertensive arterial necrosis
- Inflammatory (e.g., giant cell arteritis)
- Hemorrhage under an atherosclerotic plaque
- Associated with central retinal vein obstruction

CLINICAL SIGNS

- Visual acuity: Generally, there is a history of acute, unilateral, painless visual field loss occurring over several seconds. Approximately 10% of those affected have a history of transient visual loss (amaurosis fugax) in the affected eye prior to the central retinal arterial obstruction.

- Pupillary changes: An afferent pupillary defect may present immediately, depending on the area of distribution of the obstruction.

- Fundus changes: Three variants occur:

  ▪ Cilioretinal artery obstruction alone (Fig. 4-6): Superficial retinal whitening, usually located within the papillomacular bundle, but which may take hours to develop

  ▪ Cilioretinal artery obstruction associated with central retinal vein obstruction

  ▪ Cilioretinal artery obstruction associated with acute anterior ischemic optic neuropathy (Fig. 4-7): Must be particularly concerned about underlying giant cell arteritis

- Retinal intra-arterial emboli: Prevalence is uncertain.

  ▪ Cholesterol (Hollenhorst plaque named after Robert Hollenhorst at the Mayo Clinic): Glistening yellow and typically arises from the carotid arteries. The most likely scenario follows:

    1. Atherosclerosis causes turbulent flow.

    2. Turbulence causes damage to the carotid endothelium.

    3. Plaque is dislodged from the underlying, exposed carotid atherosclerosis. The plaque travels to lodge in the central retinal artery or branch retinal artery.

    4. A fibrin–platelet thrombus may or may not be the nidus for the development of a platelet–thrombin. Thus, a larger embolus may cause a more severe occlusion.

    5. Eventually, the endothelium repairs the damage and the plaque is not exposed to blood.

    6. Turbulence

  ▪ Calcific: Large, white plaque generally originating from the cardiac valves

  ▪ Fibrin–platelet: Longer and dull white; may originate from the carotids or cardiac valves

DIFFERENTIAL DIAGNOSIS

- Inflammatory retinitis from entities such as toxoplasmosis or cytomegalovirus. Retinal hemorrhages are typically present with the latter.

- There are also usually vitreous cells present with inflammatory conditions but not with acute cilioretinal artery obstruction.

DIAGNOSTIC EVALUATION

- Intravenous fluorescein angiography: Cilioretinal arteries normally fill with fluorescein dye during the early choroidal filling phase of a fluorescein angiogram. A cilioretinal artery obstruction typically shows nonperfusion of dye in the affected vessel through the retinal arteriovenous phase.

- Systemic workup: This is similar to that of acute central retinal artery obstruction.

  - Emboli: Carotid and cardiac

  - Inflammatory: Giant cell arteritis, Wegener's granulomatosis, polyarteritis nodosa, systemic lupus erythematosus, orbital mucormycosis, toxoplasmosis retinitis

  - Coagulopathies: Sickle cell disease, homocystinuria, lupus anticoagulant

syndrome, protein S deficiency, protein C deficiency, antithrombin III deficiency

  - Miscellaneous: Fibromuscular hyperplasia, Sydenham's chorea, Fabry's disease, migraine, Lyme disease, hypotension

PROGNOSIS AND MANAGEMENT

- With isolated cilioretinal artery obstruction, 90% of eyes return to 20/40 vision or better. With central retinal vein occlusion, 70% of eyes return to 20/40 vision or better. With anterior ischemic optic neuropathy, vision often remains counting fingers to hand motions.

- There is no consistently proven treatment to ameliorate the visual acuity. Because of the relatively good prognosis for central vision, digital massage and anterior chamber paracentesis are not typically undertaken.

- Despite the lack of an effective ocular treatment, a systemic workup should be undertaken. Although giant cell arteritis likely only accounts for 1% to 2% of cases, the possibility should be actively investigated because the fellow eye can be involved by retinal arterial obstruction within hours to days.

FIGURE 4-6. **Cilioretinal artery obstruction.** Isolated cilioretinal artery obstruction. Note the retinal whitening indicating ischemic retinal edema (inset).

FIGURE 4-7. **Cilioretinal artery obstruction and ischemic optic neuropathy.** Cilioretinal artery occlusion associated with anterior ischemic optic neuropathy. Note the associated disc edema and pallor.

BRANCH RETINAL ARTERY OBSTRUCTION (OCCLUSION)

Branch retinal artery obstruction is the acute blockage of blood flow within a branch retinal artery.

EPIDEMIOLOGY AND ETIOLOGY

- Branch retinal artery obstruction typically occurs in patients aged 65 years and older but can be seen at any age.
- It is seen in approximately 1:15,000 to 20,000 outpatient ophthalmology visits.
- The abnormality is unilateral in 99% of cases. No hereditary pattern is known.

PATHOPHYSIOLOGY

- Embolic
- Hypertensive arterial necrosis
- Inflammatory (e.g., giant cell arteritis)
- Hemorrhage under an atherosclerotic plaque

CLINICAL SIGNS

- Visual acuity: Generally, there is a history of acute, unilateral, painless visual field loss occurring over several seconds. Approximately 10% of those affected have a history of transient visual loss (amaurosis fugax) in the affected eye.
- Pupillary changes: An afferent pupillary defect may present immediately, depending on the area of distribution of the obstruction.
- Fundus changes: Superficial retinal whitening (Fig. 4-8A) can take hours to develop. Retinal intra-arterial emboli (prevalence uncertain):

  - Cholesterol (Hollenhorst plaque): Glistening yellow and typically from the carotid arteries
  - Calcific: Large, white plaque generally originating from the cardiac valves (Fig. 4-9)
  - Fibrin–platelet: Longer and dull white; may originate from the carotids or cardiac valves (see Fig. 4-8A)

DIFFERENTIAL DIAGNOSIS

- Inflammatory retinitis may occur from entities such as toxoplasmosis or cytomegalovirus. Retinal hemorrhages are typically present with the latter.
- There are also usually vitreous cells present with inflammatory conditions but not with acute branch retinal artery obstruction.

DIAGNOSTIC EVALUATION

- Intravenous fluorescein angiography: Reveals a delay in retinal arterial and venous filling in the area of obstruction versus the normal remaining fundus (see Fig. 4-8A). There may be staining of the ischemic retinal vasculature (see Fig. 4-8C).
- Systemic workup: This is similar to that of acute central retinal artery obstruction.

  - Embolic: Carotid and cardiac
  - Inflammatory: Giant cell arteritis, Wegener's granulomatosis, polyarteritis nodosa, systemic lupus erythematosus, orbital mucormycosis, toxoplasmosis retinitis
  - Coagulopathies: Sickle cell disease, homocysteinuria, lupus anticoagulant syndrome, protein S deficiency, protein C deficiency, antithrombin III deficiency
  - Miscellaneous: Fibromuscular hyperplasia, Sydenham's chorea, Fabry's disease, migraine, Lyme disease, hypotension

PROGNOSIS AND MANAGEMENT

- Most patients improve to 20/40 or better vision without treatment, although a field defect corresponding to the area of obstruction usually persists.

- There is no consistently proven treatment to ameliorate the visual acuity. Because of the relatively good prognosis for central vision,

digital massage and anterior chamber paracentesis are not typically undertaken.

- Despite the lack of an effective ocular treatment, a systemic workup should be undertaken. Although giant cell arteritis likely only accounts for 1% to 2% of cases, the possibility should be actively investigated because the fellow eye can be involved within hours to days.

FIGURE 4-8. **Branch retinal artery obstruction. A.** Retinal whitening (inset) due to branch retinal artery obstruction. Note the proximal intra-arterial platelet fibrin thrombus (*arrow*).

(*continued*)

FIGURE 4-8. (*Continued*) **Branch retinal artery obstruction. B.** Fluorescein angiogram corresponding to **A** reveals retinal arteriolar and capillary nonperfusion in the distribution of the occluded vessel. **C.** Staining of the inferotemporal branch retinal artery is present in the area of occlusion.

FIGURE 4-9. **Branch retinal artery obstruction, calcific plaque.** Intra-arterial calcific plaque (*arrow*) associated with branch retinal artery occlusion.

CENTRAL RETINAL ARTERY OBSTRUCTION (OCCLUSION)

Central retinal artery obstruction is the acute blockage of blood flow within the central retinal artery.

EPIDEMIOLOGY AND ETIOLOGY

- Central retinal artery obstruction typically occurs in patients aged 65 years and older but can be seen at any age.
- It is seen in approximately 1:10,000 outpatient ophthalmology visits.
- The abnormality is unilateral in 99% of cases.
- No hereditary pattern is known.

PATHOPHYSIOLOGY

- Embolic
- Hypertensive arterial necrosis
- Dissecting aneurysm within the central retinal artery
- Inflammatory (e.g., giant cell arteritis)
- Hemorrhage under an atherosclerotic plaque
- Vasospasm

CLINICAL SIGNS

- Visual acuity: Generally, there is a history of acute, unilateral, painless visual loss occurring over several seconds. Approximately 10% of those affected have a history of transient visual loss (amaurosis fugax) in the affected eye.
- Pupillary changes: An afferent pupillary defect is usually present immediately.

- Fundus changes
  - Superficial retinal whitening: Can take hours to develop
  - Cherry red spot in the foveola (Fig. 4-10)
  - Cilioretinal arterial sparing of central fovea (Fig. 4-11): Present in 10% of cases
  - Retinal intra-arterial emboli: Present in 20% of cases
  - Cholesterol (Hollenhorst plaque): Glistening yellow (Fig. 4-12) and typically originates from the carotid arteries
  - Calcific: Large, white plaque generally originating from the cardiac valves
  - Fibrin–platelet: Longer and dull white; may originate from the carotids or cardiac valves (see Fig. 4-8A)

DIFFERENTIAL DIAGNOSIS

- Acute ophthalmic artery obstruction (cherry red spot absent)
- Tay–Sach's disease (cherry red spot present, but in infants less than 1 year of age and with severe neurologic dysfunction)

DIAGNOSTIC EVALUATION

- Intravenous fluorescein angiography: Reveals delay in retinal arterial and venous filling (normally, the vein of the temporal vascular arcade should completely fill within 11 seconds after dye enters the corresponding retinal arteries.
- Electroretinography: Normal a-wave amplitude, but diminished b-wave amplitude.
- Systemic workup
  - Embolic: Carotid and cardiac
  - Inflammatory: Giant cell arteritis, Wegener's granulomatosis, polyarteritis nodosa, systemic lupus erythematosus, orbital mucormycosis

- Coagulopathies: Sickle cell disease, homocysteinuria, lupus anticoagulant syndrome, protein S deficiency, protein C deficiency, antithrombin III deficiency

- Miscellaneous: Fibromuscular hyperplasia, Sydenham's chorea, Fabry's disease, migraine, Lyme disease, hypotension

- Vasospastic: Migraine

PROGNOSIS AND MANAGEMENT

- The visual prognosis is typically poor, with most patients retaining counting finger to hand motions vision and a small temporal island of vision remaining. If a cilioretinal artery spares the central fovea, 80% of eyes will return to 20/20 to 20/50 vision over a period of 2 weeks. Nevertheless, in the latter instance there is typically severe visual field loss. Approximately 18% of eyes will progress to develop iris neovascularization within 4 to 6 weeks after the acute obstruction.

- There is no consistently proven treatment to ameliorate the visual acuity. Digital massage of the globe and anterior chamber paracentesis has been advocated but has minimal benefit. Treatment with fibrinolytic agents is still considered investigational.

- Despite the lack of a consistently effective ocular treatment, a systemic workup should be undertaken. Although giant cell arteritis likely only accounts for 1% to 2% of cases, the possibility should be actively investigated because the fellow eye can be involved within hours to days. In regard to systemic workup, it should be noted that patients with acute central artery obstruction have a high death rate from cardiac vascular disease.

- If iris neovascularization develops, laser panretinal photocoagulation (PRP) should be considered to help prevent neovascular glaucoma. It causes resolution of the new iris vessels in approximately two-thirds of the treated cases.

- Embolectomy has been performed with the yttrium-aluminium-garnet (YAG) by creating a hole in the artery over the laser, though the incidence of vitreous hemorrhage is high and the results variable.

FIGURE 4-10. **Acute central retinal artery occlusion.** Superficial retinal opacification is present, and a cherry red spot can be seen in the foveola. Note the segmented columns of blood in retinal arterioles (boxcarring).

FIGURE 4-11. **Central retinal artery occlusion with cilioretinal artery sparing.** Acute central retinal artery occlusion (inset) with cilioretinal arterial sparing of the foveola. Compare with Figure 4-6.

FIGURE 4-12. **Hollenhorst plaque.** Glistening cholesterol embolus (Hollenhorst plaque) within a retinal arteriole (*arrow*). These emboli typically lodge at retinal arteriolar bifurcations.

ACUTE OPHTHALMIC ARTERY OBSTRUCTION (OCCLUSION)

Acute ophthalmic artery obstruction is the acute blockage of the ophthalmic artery.

EPIDEMIOLOGY AND ETIOLOGY

• Acute ophthalmic artery obstruction occurs in approximately 1:100,000 ophthalmologic visits.

• The mean age of onset is in the sixties.

• No hereditary pattern is known.

PATHOPHYSIOLOGY

• Embolic

• Trauma

• Infectious (e.g., mucormycosis of the orbit)

• Inflammatory (e.g., collagen vascular disease, giant cell arteritis)

• Other (see causes of acute central retinal artery obstruction)

CLINICAL FEATURES

• Visual acuity: Generally, there is a history of acute, unilateral, painless visual loss occurring over a period ranging from seconds. The visual acuity is no light perception in 90% of cases.

• Pupillary changes: An afferent pupillary defect is present.

• Fundus changes: Superficial retinal whitening in the posterior pole occurs, often more pronounced than with acute central retinal artery obstruction because the retinal pigment epithelium may be opacified as well with acute ophthalmic artery obstruction (Fig. 4-13A). The presence of a cherry red spot in the foveola is variable; one-third of the patients have none, one-third have a mild cherry red spot, and one-third have a prominent cherry red spot.

• The presence of retinal arterial emboli is variable. "Salt and pepper" retinal pigment epithelial changes occur in the posterior pole and elsewhere within weeks after the acute obstruction. The pigment epithelial changes do not occur secondary to central retinal artery obstruction alone.

DIFFERENTIAL DIAGNOSIS

• Refer to Table 4-1.

DIAGNOSTIC EVALUATION

• Intravenous fluorescein angiography

   ▪ Delay in choroidal filling: The choroid should be completely filled within

TABLE 4-1. Differential Diagnosis of Acute Ophthalmic Artery Obstruction

	Central Retinal Artery Obstruction	Ophthalmic Artery Obstruction
Vision	Finger counting—hand motions	No light perception
Fundus	Retinal opacification with cherry red spot	Marked opacification ± cherry red spot
Fluorescein angiography	Delayed retinal vascular filling	Delayed choroidal and retinal vascular filling
Electroretinography	Decreased b-wave	Decreased a- and b-waves

5 seconds after the first appearance of fluorescein dye within it (Fig. 4-13B).

- ▪ Delayed retinal arterial and venous filling.

- ▪ Late focal or diffuse staining of the retinal pigment epithelium due to choroidal ischemia.

- Electroretinography: Decreased or absent a-wave (outer layer retinal ischemia) and b-wave (inner layer retinal ischemia) amplitudes.

- Systemic workup: This is similar to that of acute central retinal artery obstruction.

  - ▪ Embolic: Carotid and cardiac

  - ▪ Inflammatory: Giant cell arteritis, Wegener's granulomatosis, polyarteritis nodosa, systemic lupus erythematosus, orbital mucormycosis, toxoplasmosis retinitis.

  - ▪ Coagulopathies: Sickle cell disease, homocysteinuria, lupus anticoagulant syndrome, protein S deficiency, protein C deficiency, antithrombin III deficiency

  - ▪ Miscellaneous: Fibromuscular hyperplasia, Sydenham's chorea, Fabry's disease, migraine, Lyme disease, hypotension

- The most common etiology is as an iatrogenic sequela of retrobulbar injection.

PROGNOSIS AND MANAGEMENT

- Although spontaneous reversal can rarely occur, the long-term vision in most cases is usually light perception to no light perception. There is no proven treatment to ameliorate the visual acuity. Despite the lack of an effective ocular treatment, a systemic workup should be undertaken.

- The patient should be observed regularly for the first several months for the development of iris neovascularization. Laser PRP should be considered if iris neovascularization develops (the incidence of development of iris neovascularization is unknown).

FIGURE 4-13. **Acute ophthalmic artery obstruction. A.** Marked retinal whitening is present, and a cherry red spot is absent. The visual acuity was no light perception. **B.** Fluorescein angiogram corresponding to **A.** At 116 seconds after injection, there is no dye within the retinal vessels and the majority of the choroid. Peripapillary staining is present, presumably due to collaterals between episcleral vessels and the choroidal circulation.

COMBINED CENTRAL RETINAL ARTERY AND VEIN OBSTRUCTION (OCCLUSION)

Combined central retinal artery and vein obstruction is the acute blockage of both the central retinal artery and the central retinal vein.

EPIDEMIOLOGY AND ETIOLOGY

- The prevalence is uncertain.
- No hereditary pattern is known.

PATHOPHYSIOLOGY

- The disease process is uncertain; blockage of both the central retinal artery and the central retinal vein has been shown in one case.

CLINICAL SIGNS

- Visual acuity: Generally, there is a history of acute or subacute, unilateral, painless visual field loss occurring over a period ranging from seconds to days.
- Pupillary changes: An afferent pupillary defect is typically present.
- Fundus changes (Fig. 4-14)
  - Superficial retinal whitening in the posterior pole
  - Cherry red spot in the foveola
  - Dilated, tortuous retinal veins

- Retinal hemorrhages
- Macular edema

DIFFERENTIAL DIAGNOSIS

- Inflammatory retinitis from cytomegalovirus
- Central retinal vein obstruction (no cherry red spot is present)

DIAGNOSTIC EVALUATION

- Intravenous fluorescein angiography: Reveals a delay in retinal arterial and venous filling in the area of obstruction versus the normal remaining fundus. Severe retinal capillary nonperfusion is often present.
- Systemic workup: This is similar to that of acute central retinal artery obstruction.
  - Embolic: Carotid and cardiac
  - Inflammatory: Giant cell arteritis, Wegener's granulomatosis, polyarteritis nodosa, systemic lupus erythematosus, orbital mucormycosis, toxoplasmosis retinitis
  - Coagulopathies: Sickle cell disease, homocysteinuria, lupus anticoagulant syndrome, protein S deficiency, protein C deficiency, antithrombin III deficiency
  - Miscellaneous: Fibromuscular hyperplasia, Sydenham's chorea, Fabry's disease, migraine, Lyme disease, hypotension
- The most common etiology is as a sequela of retrobulbar injection.

PROGNOSIS AND MANAGEMENT

- Although there are exceptions, the vision most often remains in the counting fingers to light perception range. Approximately 80% of eyes will progress to iris neovascularization at a mean time of approximately 6 weeks after the obstruction.

- There is no proven treatment to ameliorate the visual acuity. Despite the lack of an effective ocular treatment, a systemic workup should be undertaken. The patient should be followed regularly for the first several months for the development of iris neovascularization.

- Laser PRP should be considered if iris neovascularization develops.

- If the visual acuity is counting fingers or worse, PRP can be considered prior to the development of iris neovascularization.

FIGURE 4-14. **Combined central retinal artery and central retinal vein occlusion.** The retinal veins are dilated and tortuous, retinal hemorrhages are present, and a cherry red spot due to superficial retinal opacification can be seen.

OCULAR ISCHEMIC SYNDROME

Ocular ischemic syndrome describes ocular symptoms and signs attributable to marked carotid or ophthalmic artery obstruction. Alternative nomenclatures include venous stasis retinopathy, ischemic ocular inflammation, and ischemic oculopathy.

EPIDEMIOLOGY AND ETIOLOGY

- Approximately 2000 cases occur in the United States per year.
- The entity is unilateral in 80% of cases and bilateral in 20%.
- It occurs in approximately 5% of patients with carotid artery obstruction and is not usually seen in those under the age of 50 years.
- The mean age is 65 years.
- No hereditary pattern is known.

PATHOPHYSIOLOGY

- Disease involves blockage of the carotid or ophthalmic artery, or both. No flow disturbance occurs until there is 70% obstruction. With 90% obstruction, perfusion pressure in the central retinal artery decreases by 50%. Half of the cases have a 100% ipsilateral common or internal carotid artery obstruction. Causes include:
  - Atherosclerosis (over 90% of cases)
  - Giant cell arteritis

CLINICAL FEATURES

- Symptoms and signs
  - Vision: Decreases over a period of weeks to months, although in 12% there is acute visual loss associated with a cherry red spot.

  - Periorbital pain: "Ocular angina" is present in about 40% of cases and is described as a dull ache.
  - Prolonged visual recovery time after exposure to bright light.
  - Pupillary changes: An afferent pupillary defect is typically present.
- Anterior segment
  - Iris neovascularization (67%)
  - Anterior chamber cells (20%)
- Posterior segment
  - Narrowed retinal arteries in most cases
  - Dilated, but not tortuous, retinal veins (**Fig. 4-15A**) in most cases
  - Microaneurysms (see **Fig. 4-15C**) in most cases (posterior pole or peripheral, or both)
  - Retinal dot and blot hemorrhages (80% of eyes)
  - Neovascularization of the optic disc and/or retina (35%)
  - Superficial retinal whitening in the posterior pole (12%)
  - Macular edema (see **Fig. 4-15B**) (11%)
  - Spontaneous retinal arterial pulsations (4%)
- Associated systemic abnormalities
  - Systemic arterial hypertension (65%)
  - Cardiac disease (50%)
  - Diabetes mellitus (50%)
  - Previous stroke (20%)
  - Severe peripheral vascular disease (20%)

DIFFERENTIAL DIAGNOSIS

- Central retinal vein obstruction typically has tortuous retinal veins, as well as more retinal hemorrhages and macular edema than the ocular ischemic syndrome. Light digital pressure on the lid, or minimal pressure with ophthalmodynamometry, will induce retinal arterial pulsations with the ocular ischemic syndrome, whereas substantial pressure is required with central retinal vein occlusion. Also consider:

- Diabetic retinopathy
- Radiation retinopathy

DIAGNOSTIC EVALUATION

- Intravenous fluorescein angiography: Delay in choroidal filling (**Fig. 4-16**) occurs in 60% of cases. Delayed retinal arterial and venous filling (see **Fig. 4-16**) occurs in 95% of cases. Late retinal vascular staining, more pronounced of the retinal arteries (**Fig. 4-17**), occurs in 85% of cases.

- Electroretinography: Decreased or absent a-wave (outer layer retinal ischemia) and b-wave (inner layer retinal ischemia) amplitudes are seen.

- Systemic workup: Carotid noninvasive studies have approximately 90% chance of detecting carotid stenosis of 50% or more. Carotid arteriography or magnetic resonance angiography (MRA) is performed if carotid noninvasive studies are ambiguous or if carotid artery surgery is being considered.

PROGNOSIS

- Ocular: Seventy-five percent of eyes will progress to counting fingers of worse vision within 1 year after diagnosis.

- Systemic: There is a 40% 5-year mortality, with cardiac disease as the most common cause of death.

MANAGEMENT

- Laser PRP is performed if there is iris neovascularization and the anterior chamber angle is open. PRP induces regression of iris new vessels in 36% of cases. The patient should be evaluated for possible carotid endarterectomy. In surgical candidates, 33% demonstrate improved vision, 33% demonstrate stabilized vision, and 33% progress to lose vision despite endarterectomy surgery.

- If the carotid artery is 100% obstructed, endarterectomy is not of benefit; neither is extracranial to intracranial (e.g., superficial temporal to middle cerebral) bypass. Remember not to ignore the cardiac status, because cardiac disease is the leading cause of death.

- Endarterectomy is indicated for symptomatic patients (those with amaurosis fugax, transient ischemic attack, or nondisabling stroke), and those with 70% to 99% ipsilateral carotid stenosis (**Table 4-2**). Antiplatelet therapy is indicated for those who are symptomatic and have less than 70% stenosis.

- Carotid stenting can also be considered in select cases.

TABLE 4-2. Outcomes After Treatment of Symptomatic Patients with High-grade Carotid Artery Stenosis

	Endarterectomy	Antiplatelet Agent
Perioperative mortality	2%	1%
Severe stroke by 2 years	9%	26%

Data from the North American Symptomatic Carotid Endarterectomy Trial (NASCET).

FIGURE 4-15. **Ocular ischemic syndrome. A.** The retinal veins are slightly dilated, but not tortuous, and the retinal arteries are narrowed. A few retinal hemorrhages are noted in the macula. **B.** Fluorescein angiogram corresponding to **A.** Hyperfluorescence of the optic disc and macular edema are prominent.

(*continued*)

FIGURE 4-15. (*Continued*) **Ocular ischemic syndrome. C.** Fluorescein angiogram in an eye with ocular ischemic syndrome demonstrating pinpoint foci of hyperfluorescence due to microaneurysms in the midperipheral fundus.

FIGURE 4-16. Ocular ischemic syndrome. Fluorescein angiogram revealing delayed retinal arterial and choroidal vascular filling in an ocular ischemic syndrome eye. Note the abnormal leading edge of fluorescein dye in the retinal arteriole (*arrow*).

FIGURE 4-17. **Ocular ischemic syndrome.** Late-phase fluorescein angiogram demonstrating retinal vascular staining in an ocular ischemic syndrome eye.

BRANCH RETINAL VEIN OBSTRUCTION (OCCLUSION)

Branch retinal vein obstruction is the acute blockage of blood flow within a branch retinal vein.

EPIDEMIOLOGY AND ETIOLOGY

- Branch retinal vein obstruction typically occurs in patients aged 65 years and older but can be seen at any age. The Beaver Dam Eye Study noted a prevalence of 0.6% and a 5-year incidence of 0.6% as well. No hereditary pattern is known.

PATHOPHYSIOLOGY

- Branch retinal vein occlusion typically occurs at a retinal arteriovenous crossing. Impingement of the branch retinal artery on the branch retinal vein is believed to cause turbulent flow, leading to endothelial cell damage and predisposing to thrombus formation within the branch retinal vein.
- When the branch retinal vein occlusion does not occur at an arteriovenous crossing, an inflammatory cause, such as from sarcoidosis, should be considered.

CLINICAL SIGNS

- Visual acuity: Generally, there is a history of unilateral, painless visual loss occurring over a period of days.
- Pupillary changes: An afferent pupillary defect may be present, depending on the size of the venous occlusion and the degree of retinal ischemia.
- Anterior segment changes: Iris neovascularization has been observed to develop in

5% to 10% of hemispheric retinal vein occlusions and 1% to 2% of branch retinal vein obstructions.

- Posterior segment changes: Retinal venous engorgement and tortuosity, as well as retinal hemorrhages and edema, are typically present within the distribution of the occluded vessel (Fig. 4-18A). Macular branch (twig) vein occlusions may be clinically subtle with minimal hemorrhage, telangiectasia, or macular edema.
- Neovascularization of the optic disc or retina, or both, can develop months to years after the occlusion. Vitreous traction on retinal or optic disc neovascularization may lead to vitreous hemorrhage with or without traction retinal detachment.

DIFFERENTIAL DIAGNOSIS

- Retinal cavernous hemangioma can occasionally mimic the appearance of a branch retinal vein occlusion.

DIAGNOSTIC EVALUATION

- Intravenous fluorescein angiography: Reveals a delay in retinal arterial and venous filling in the distribution of the obstructed vessel. Retinal capillary nonperfusion may be present (Fig. 4-18B).
- Systemic workup: Includes an evaluation for systemic arterial hypertension and increased body mass. A history of glaucoma has also been associated with branch retinal vein occlusion.

PROGNOSIS AND MANAGEMENT

Laser Photocoagulation for Macular Edema
- The mean resultant visual acuity in eyes with untreated branch retinal vein occlusion

in the Branch Vein Occlusion Study is 20/70. In eyes that are candidates for grid laser photocoagulation for macular edema, the mean visual result is 20/40 to 20/50.

• According to the Branch Vein Occlusion Study, laser grid photocoagulation for visual loss due to macular edema can be considered for eyes with branch retinal occlusion that meet the following criteria:

▪ Visual acuity of 20/40 to 20/200

▪ Intact perifoveal capillaries with fluorescein angiography

▪ Resolution of the majority of intraretinal blood

Ranibizumab Therapy for Macular Edema, the Primary Treatment

• The BRAVO Clinical Trial demonstrated that the mean vision in a cohort of untreated patients with branch retinal vein occlusion was approximately 20/70, while the cohort treated with intravitreal ranibizumab once a month for 6 months resulted in a mean visual acuity of approximately 20/30. Unlike the case with laser photocoagulation therapy, ranibizumab therapy does not leave visual field defects (which tend to enlarge considerably over years) within the macular region. Ranibizumab should be considered the primary treatment therapy for the treatment of macular edema associated with branch retinal vein occlusion.

Sector Laser PRP

• If posterior segment neovascularization develops, sector laser PRP in the distribution of the obstructed branch retinal vein should be considered. This therapy reduces the incidence of subsequent vitreous hemorrhage from approximately 60% to 30%.

• If iris neovascularization develops, sector laser PRP should be considered to help prevent neovascular glaucoma.

• The BRAVO study, in which intravitreal 0.5 mg ranibizumab injections were given monthly for 6 months, patients gained almost three lines of vision, meaning they saw twice as well as sham therapy. The near vision without ranibizumab at 6 months was 20/70 at baseline improving to 20/32 with ranibizumab.

FIGURE 4-18. Branch retinal vein occlusion. A. Retinal hemorrhages and cotton-wool spots are present in the distribution of the occluded vessel (inset). **B.** Fluorescein angiogram corresponding to **A.** Retinal capillary nonperfusion is present in the distribution of the occluded vessel. **C.** Optical coherence tomography in eye with a branch retinal vein occlusion demonstrating macular edema.

CENTRAL RETINAL VEIN OBSTRUCTION (OCCLUSION)

Central retinal vein obstruction is blockage of blood flow within the central retinal vein.

EPIDEMIOLOGY AND ETIOLOGY

- Central retinal vein obstruction typically occurs in patients aged 65 years and older but can be seen at any age.
- In the Beaver Dam Eye Study, the prevalence was 0.1% and the 5-year incidence was 0.2%.
- Bilaterality eventually occurs in approximately 10% of cases, more commonly in those with underlying systemic abnormalities.
- No hereditary pattern is known.

PATHOPHYSIOLOGY

- Intravenous thrombus at or near the lamina cribrosa is seen in eyes with central retinal vein obstruction studied histopathologically. Impingement of the central retinal artery on the central retinal vein is believed to cause turbulence and subsequent endothelial damage, which predisposes to thrombus formation.
- Increased intraocular pressure may also predispose to central retinal vein obstruction by theoretically bowing the lamina cribrosa posteriorly, leading to turbulence, endothelial damage, and thrombus formation.

CLINICAL SIGNS

- Visual acuity: Generally, there is a history of unilateral, painless visual loss occurring over hours to days or weeks. Nonischemic central retinal vein occlusions (**Fig. 4-19**) typically are associated with vision of 20/200 or better, whereas ischemic central retinal vein obstructions (**Fig. 4-20A–E**) are associated with vision of counting fingers or worse.
    - Approximately 20% of eyes with nonischemic central retinal vein occlusion will eventually progress to the ischemic variant.
- Pupillary changes: An afferent pupillary defect may be present, increasing in severity as the visual acuity decreases and the degree of ischemia increases.
- Anterior segment changes: Iris neovascularization (rubeosis iridis) develops in approximately 20% of cases at a mean time of 3 to 5 months after the obstruction.
- Posterior segment changes
    - Dilated, tortuous retinal veins
    - Retinal hemorrhages, most pronounced in the posterior pole
    - Retinal edema, most pronounced in the macula
    - Neovascularization of the optic disc or retina, or both, or optic disc collaterals (**Fig. 4-20F**); may develop months after the obstruction

DIFFERENTIAL DIAGNOSIS

- Differential diagnosis includes ocular ischemic syndrome (**Table 4-3**). Diabetic retinopathy can also mimic central retinal vein obstruction, but the former is typically bilateral, has prominent hard exudates (rare in central retinal vein obstruction) and many more microaneurysms than with central retinal vein obstruction.

DIAGNOSTIC EVALUATION

- Intravenous fluorescein angiography reveals delay in retinal venous filling and

TABLE 4-3. Differential Diagnosis of Central Retinal Vein Obstruction

	Central Retinal Vein Obstruction	Ocular Ischemic Syndrome
Vision	20/20—hand motions	20/20—no light perception
Iris neovascularization	20%	67%
Retinal hemorrhages	Mild to severe	Mild
Retinal venous tortuosity	Usually present	Absent
Macular edema	Mild to severe	Mild
Fluorescein angiography		
Choroidal filling	Normal	Delayed
Retinal AV transit	Delayed	Delayed
Late arterial staining	Absent	Present

AV, arteriovenous.

intraretinal leakage of dye, most prominent in the macula, as the study progresses. Increasing areas of retinal capillary nonperfusion can be seen in more ischemic cases. When the retinal capillary nonperfusion (in seven fundus photographic fields) exceeds 75 disc areas, the incidence of development of iris neovascularization rises to more than 50%.

- Electroretinography: Normal a-wave amplitude, but diminished b-wave amplitude, occurs as ischemia increases.

- Systemic workup
  - Systemic arterial hypertension
  - Diabetes mellitus
  - Hyperviscosity syndromes (e.g., polycythemia vera, Waldenstrom's macroglobulinemia, plasma cell dyscrasias such as multiple myeloma)
  - Hyperlipidemias
  - Inflammatory or infectious (e.g., sarcoidosis, systemic lupus erythematosus, syphilis)
  - Hypercoagulability states (e.g., lupus anticoagulant syndrome, protein S deficiency, protein C deficiency, antithrombin III deficiency, hyperhomocysteinemia)

PROGNOSIS AND MANAGEMENT

- Until the use of intravitreal ranibizumab injections for the treatment of the macular edema associated with central retinal vein occlusion, there was no effective intervention. The CRUISE Clinical Trial demonstrated that 6-monthly intravitreal injections of 0.5mg ranibizumab resulted in a visual acuity of 20/32, while the untreated cohort had a mean visual acuity of 20/63.

- According to the guidelines of the Central Retinal Vein Occlusion Study, if any anterior chamber angle neovascularization or 2 clock hours or more of iris neovascularization develops, laser PRP should be considered to help prevent neovascular glaucoma.

FIGURE 4-19. **Nonischemic central retinal vein occlusion.** Note the retinal hemorrhages in all four quadrants around the optic disc. The visual acuity in the eye was 20/50.

FIGURE 4-20. Ischemic central retinal occlusion. A. Retinal hemorrhage, diffuse retinal edema, and numerous cotton-wool spots are present. The visual acuity was hand motions. **B.** Fluorescein angiogram corresponding to **A.** Areas of marked retinal capillary nonperfusion and macular edema are present. Some of the areas of hypofluorescence correspond to retinal hemorrhages.

(*continued*)

FIGURE 4-20. (*Continued*) **Ischemic central retinal occlusion. C.** Retinal hemorrhage, retinal venous tortuosity, diffuse macular edema, and markedly narrowed retinal arterioles are present. **D.** Fluorescein angiogram corresponding to **C.** Delayed retinal venous filling and retinal telangiectasia are noted. There is marked hypofluorescence from retinal ischemia and blockage from retinal hemorrhages.

(*continued*)

FIGURE 4-20. (*Continued*) **Ischemic central retinal occlusion. E.** Fluorescein angiogram corresponding to **C.** There is widespread macular ischemia. **F.** Optic disc collaterals shunting retinal venous blood to the choroidal circulation may be noted on the optic disc.

RETINAL ARTERIAL MACROANEURYSM

First described in 1973, retinal arterial macroaneurysm is characterized by the presence of vascular dilation or outpouching of a retinal artery or arteriole.

EPIDEMIOLOGY

- Retinal arterial macroaneurysms occur as isolated phenomena in two-thirds of the cases. About one-third of the cases are seen in conjunction with retinal venous obstructions.
- Ten percent of cases are bilateral.

PATHOPHYSIOLOGY

- The aneurysms are believed to be clinically similar in size (300 μm) to the intracerebral variant, although no association with intracerebral aneurysms has been convincingly demonstrated.
- They can occur as saccular dilations within the vessel or as outpouchings from the vessel.
- About three quarters of cases are associated with systemic arterial hypertension.

CLINICAL SIGNS

- The entity is typically unilateral and isolated. Pulsations of the macroaneurysm are occasionally seen. The two most common variants of presentation are as follows:

  - Acute hemorrhage may develop in the subretinal space, retinal or preretinal region if the macroaneurysms ruptures. A multilevel hemorrhage should arouse suspicion of the presence of a macroaneurysm. A white or yellow spot (the aneurysm) is often present centrally within the hemorrhage (**Fig. 4-21**). Recurrent bleeding is extremely unusual.

  - Retinal edema may be the presenting sign when chronic leakage of plasma encroaches upon the fovea. In this instance, lipid exudation is also often present.

- In approximately 4% of cases, a retinal arterial obstruction distal to the macroaneurysm is seen at the time of presentation.

DIFFERENTIAL DIAGNOSIS

- The abnormality is relatively unique in appearance. Aneurysmal abnormalities associated with Coats' disease can occasionally cause bleeding seen with retinal arterial macroaneurysms, but with Coats' disease there are typically multiple aneurysmal arterial or venous dilations, or both.

- The presence of multiple, bilateral arterial aneurysmal abnormalities occurring principally at arterial bifurcations has been described with the disorder, termed idiopathic retinal vasculitis, aneurysms, and neuroretinitis (IRVAN).

DIAGNOSTIC EVALUATION

- Intravenous fluorescein angiography reveals hyperfluorescence corresponding to the macroaneurysm (**Fig. 4-21B**). Vascular telangiectasias surrounding the aneurysmal abnormality may be present.

PROGNOSIS AND MANAGEMENT

- The visual prognosis depends on whether bleeding involves the central macular region. In such instances, vision can be reduced to counting fingers or worse. Spontaneous improvement can occur, particularly when the blood is located superficially within the retina. Involvement of the macula by edema can lead to visual loss, typically ranging from 20/25 to 20/200.

- The bleeding associated with macroaneurysms is not typically treated. It is usually a one-time event, and visual improvement can occur when the hemorrhage is located primarily within the superficial layers of the retina.

- Although there are no randomized clinical studies addressing the issue, most retinal experts recommend treating the macroaneurysms when there is involvement of the central fovea by retinal edema or hard exudation, or both. Treatment is given using 200- to 500-μm spot size, light argon laser burns to the aneurysm and the retina surrounding the abnormality.

  - In approximately 16% of cases, treatment leads to a retinal arterial obstruction distal to the aneurysm. Thus, treatment of aneurysms that could lead to an arterial obstruction involving the central macula should be undertaken with caution.

  - In a cross-sectional study, 4% of eyes presented with a branch retinal artery occlusion distal to the macroaneurysm.

FIGURE 4-21. Retinal arterial macroaneurysm associated with yellowed blood. A. The blood superiorly is superficial to the retinal vessels (preretinal), whereas inferiorly it is located in the subretinal space. The yellow macroaneurysm (*arrow*) is present along the course of the retinal artery. **B.** Fluorescein angiogram corresponding to **A.** The aneurysm is hyperfluorescent and located along the inferotemporal retinal artery.

PARAFOVEAL TELANGIECTASIS

Parafoveal (juxtafoveal) telangiectasis is a retinal vascular entity characterized by the presence of incompetent retinal capillaries in the foveal region of one or both eyes.

EPIDEMIOLOGY AND ETIOLOGY

- Group 1 parafoveal telangiectasis has been associated with an abnormal glucose tolerance in more than 30% of cases. Group 2 parafoveal telangiectasis has been associated with an abnormal glucose tolerance test in more than 60% of cases. The incidence of parafoveal telangiectasis is uncertain. There is no known hereditary pattern.

PATHOPHYSIOLOGY

- Histopathology has shown thickening of the walls of the retinal capillaries by a deposition of basement membrane. The changes are similar to those seen with diabetic retinopathy.

CLINICAL SIGNS

- The entity is stratified into three variants:
  - Group 1: Unilateral parafoveal telangiectasis
  - Group 2: Bilateral parafoveal telangiectasis
  - Group 3: Bilateral occlusive parafoveal telangiectasis alone or associated with central nervous system occlusive vasculitis
- There is typically a blunted foveal reflex with localized retinal thickening most pronounced in the temporal fovea. A grayish macular reflex may be observed clinically and highlighted with red-free photography. Retinal pigment epithelial hyperplasia, most prominent in the temporal fovea, can be seen in the later stages, as can right-angle venules diving into the outer retina. Yellow intraretinal crystals in the fovea are also seen in some cases (Fig. 4-22A). Despite the retinal thickening, the retinal cystoid changes often seen with diabetic retinopathy or retinal vein obstruction are not usually present with parafoveal telangiectasis.

- In approximately 5% of patients, choroidal neovascularization can develop in the region of the telangiectatic retinal vessels.

DIFFERENTIAL DIAGNOSIS

- Diabetic retinopathy
- Radiation retinopathy
- Carotid obstructive disease (ocular ischemic syndrome)
- Twig retinal vein obstruction
- Coats' disease
- Macular edema associated with the Irvine–Gass syndrome
- Macular edema associated with uveitis
- The appearance of temporal foveal leakage with fluorescein angiography is very helpful for making the diagnosis of parafoveal telangiectasis. In contrast to the Irvine–Gass syndrome (macular edema after cataract surgery) or uveitis associated with macular edema, the optic disc is not usually hyperfluorescent in eyes with parafoveal telangiectasis.

DIAGNOSTIC EVALUATION

- The ophthalmoscopic diagnosis is often difficult. Intravenous fluorescein angiography is often required to make the diagnosis. There is characteristic intraretinal leakage of dye located primarily in the temporal macula (Fig. 4-22B).

● In the group 3 variant, areas of retinal capillary dropout can be seen in the foveal region.

PROGNOSIS AND MANAGEMENT

● When patients first present, the visual acuity is often only mildly decreased to the 20/20 to 20/30 range. Over the years, the vision can decrease dramatically to legal blindness. When abrupt loss of vision is present, the possibility of an associated choroidal neovascular membrane should be considered.

● Laser photocoagulation has not been shown to be of benefit for the treatment of parafoveal telangiectasis. Laser therapy may be of benefit in treating the choroidal neovascularization associated with parafoveal telangiectasis. Patients should be made aware of the strong association between an abnormal glucose tolerance test and parafoveal telangiectasis, especially the group 2 variant.

FIGURE 4-22. **Group 2 parafoveal telangiectasis. A.** The temporal foveal retina is thickened, and crystalline deposits are present in this area as well. The visual acuity in the eye was 20/100. Inset highlights telangiectatic changes.

(continued)

FIGURE 4-22. (*Continued*) **Group 2 parafoveal telangiectasis. B.** Early-phase fluorescein angiogram corresponding to **A.** Telangiectatic retinal vascular changes are present surrounding the foveal avascular zone. **C.** Late-phase fluorescein angiogram corresponding to **A.** Intraretinal leakage of dye is present in the vicinity of the telangiectatic changes in the temporal fovea.

SICKLE CELL RETINOPATHY

Sickle cell retinopathy describes the fundus changes associated with sickle cell hemoglobinopathies.

EPIDEMIOLOGY

- Approximately 10% of the U.S. population have any form of sickle hemoglobin; 0.4% have hemoglobin SS, 0.2% have hemoglobin SC, and 0.03% have sickle cell thalassemia (SThal).
- Proliferative sickle retinopathy has been noted to occur in Jamaican individuals with sickle hemoglobinopathy in the following percentages: SS, 3%; SC, 33%; and SThal, 14%.

PATHOPHYSIOLOGY

- Sickled red blood cells cause obstruction within the retinal vasculature. Multiple hemoglobin variants have been described, along with their genetic changes. Although SS disease is associated with more severe systemic disease, SC disease causes more advanced ocular disease.

CLINICAL SIGNS

Nonproliferative Manifestations

- Salmon patch hemorrhage: An oval-shaped area of intraretinal or preretinal blood believed to occur secondary to an obstructed retinal arteriole, which subsequently ruptures.
- Iridescent spot: A small retinoschisis cavity within the superficial retina that can occur as a salmon patch resolves. It is filled with hemosiderin-laden macrophages.
- Black sunburst lesion (Fig. 4-23): An oval or round collection of retinal pigment epithelial cells that are believed to develop from a salmon patch hemorrhage that has dissected into the subretinal space or from a focal choroidal occlusion.

Proliferative Changes

- Five stages have been described.
  - Stage I: Peripheral retinal arteriolar occlusions
  - Stage II: Peripheral retinal arteriovenous anastomoses
  - Stage III: Peripheral retinal neovascularization ("sea fans") (Fig. 4-24A)
  - Stage IV: Vitreous hemorrhage
  - Stage V: Rhegmatogenous or traction retinal detachment, or both

DIFFERENTIAL DIAGNOSIS

- Eales' disease
- Proliferative diabetic retinopathy
- Radiation retinopathy
- Retinal vein occlusion
- Sarcoidosis

DIAGNOSTIC EVALUATION

- A history of sickle cell disease may be elicited, and thus a sickle cell prep or hemoglobin electrophoresis should be considered when characteristic findings are noted.
- The disease is diagnosed by its clinical appearance. Intravenous fluorescein angiography reveals retinal capillary nonperfusion adjacent and peripheral to areas of peripheral retinal neovascularization (Fig. 4-24).

PROGNOSIS AND MANAGEMENT

- The visual prognosis is often relatively good unless the sequelae of proliferative sickle disease (vitreous hemorrhage or retinal detachment, or both) develop.

- Treatment is not indicated for the nonproliferative changes of sickling hemoglobinopathies. When peripheral retinal neovascularization is present, full scatter laser photocoagulation to the retina peripheral to the neovascularization has been shown to reduce the incidence of subsequent vitreous hemorrhage. Many have advocated treating the peripheral retina for 360 degrees.

- Para plana vitrectomy can be of benefit for chronic vitreous hemorrhage. Vitrectomy, with or without scleral buckling, may be of benefit for the repair of retinal detachment.

FIGURE 4-23. **Sickle cell retinopathy, "black sunburst lesion."** Small, black sunburst lesion (inset) in an eye with sickle cell retinopathy. There is a sclerotic retinal vessel leading to ischemic peripheral retina inferiorly.

FIGURE 4-24. Stage 3 proliferative sickle cell retinopathy. A. Orange "sea fans," or areas of peripheral retinal neovascularization, are present at the juncture of perfused and ischemic peripheral retina. **B.** Fluorescein angiogram corresponding to (**A**) at 29 seconds after injection. The sea fans are hyperfluorescent, and retinal capillary nonperfusion is visible adjacent to them on the left side of the photo.

(continued)

FIGURE 4-24. (*Continued*) **Stage 3 proliferative sickle cell retinopathy. C.** Late-phase fluorescein angiogram showing marked leakage of fluorescein dye into the vitreous from the retinal sea fan neovascularization.

RADIATION RETINOPATHY

R adiation retinopathy refers to damage induced to the retina or optic nerve, or both, by external beam irradiation (teletherapy) or by localized irradiation (brachytherapy). The optic nerve changes are referred to as radiation optic neuropathy.

EPIDEMIOLOGY AND ETIOLOGY

- Damage from external beam irradiation often occurs from irradiation to structures adjacent to the eyes (brain, oropharynx, etc.). Typically, a minimum dose of 1500 cGy (centigray) of external beam irradiation is required to induce retinopathy. The mean dose is about 5000 cGy. At a dose of 7000 to 8000 cGy, 85% of eyes will develop radiation retinopathy. Fraction sizes of more than 200 per day appear to amplify the chances of radiation damage. For 60Co brachytherapy, a minimum of 20,000 cGy to the tumor base is necessary to induce radiation changes, with the average dose over 30,000 cGy.

PATHOPHYSIOLOGY

- Radiation retinopathy and optic neuropathy are caused primarily by damage to the vasculature of the respective structures.

CLINICAL SIGNS

- Radiation changes usually occur at a mean time of 12 to 18 months after the termination of radiation, with a range from 1 month to 7 years. The condition can be unilateral or bilateral, depending on the fields included in the irradiation.
- Visual acuity is variable, depending on the degree of damage to the retinal or optic nerve vasculature.

- The retinal changes (Fig. 4-25) are characterized by the presence of cotton-wool spots, retinal hemorrhages, and hard exudation. Neovascularization of the optic disc or retina, or both, can develop as well. Optic nerve changes are characterized by disc edema, at times in conjunction with peripapillary subretinal fluid and lipid exudation (Fig. 4-26). Retinopathy and optic neuropathy can occur concomitantly or separately.
- The fundus findings with brachytherapy are similar to those with teletherapy (Fig. 4-27), although hard exudation tends to be a more prominent feature with brachytherapy (Fig. 4-28).

DIFFERENTIAL DIAGNOSIS

- Radiation retinopathy can closely mimic diabetic retinopathy. There are usually more microaneurysms present with diabetic retinopathy than with radiation retinopathy. Key to the diagnosis of radiation is the elicitation of a history of radiation to or around the eyes.

DIAGNOSTIC EVALUATION

- Intravenous fluorescein angiography reveals retinal capillary dropout, retinal vascular telangiectases, and late leakage of dye from the damaged vessels.

PROGNOSIS AND MANAGEMENT

- The visual prognosis depends on the dose of radiation received. The presence of chemotherapy, systemic arterial hypertension, diabetic retinopathy, and other diseases that can damage the retinal vasculature appear to be additive to the radiation damage.
- With brachytherapy for choroidal melanoma, about two-thirds of the eyes have

20/200 vision or better at 2 to 3 years after treatment.

- Approximately 25% untreated eyes with radiation retinopathy from external beam irradiation progress to develop iris neo-vascularization of the iris and neovascular glaucoma.

- Macular edema can be treated with focal laser therapy in a fashion similar to the treatment of clinically significant macular edema in the Early Treatment Diabetic Retinopathy Study. Laser PRP is indicated when neovascularization of the iris or posterior segment neovascularization develops.

- There is no known effective treatment for radiation optic neuropathy, but spontaneous improvement of vision occurs in about 20% of cases.

FIGURE 4-25. Radiation retinopathy after teletherapy. A. Cotton-wool spots and small retinal hemorrhage are present in the posterior pole. **B.** Fluorescein angiogram corresponding to **A** at 25 seconds after injection. The cotton-wool spots are hypofluorescent. Note the radiation-induced capillary telangiectasia at the fovea and below the inferior retinal vascular arcade where capillary nonperfusion is noted.

(*continued*)

FIGURE 4-25. (*Continued*) **Radiation retinopathy after teletherapy. C.** Fluorescein angiogram corresponding to **A** at 375 seconds after injections. The cotton-wool spots are now more hyperfluorescent due to leakage of dye from the retina at their border.

FIGURE 4-26. **Radiation optic neuropathy after teletherapy.** The optic disc is swollen and surrounded by peripapillary lipid exudates and subretinal fluid.

FIGURE 4-27. **Radiation retinopathy following brachytherapy for a choroidal melanoma.** Cotton-wool spots are present in the peripapillary region.

FIGURE 4-28. **Radiation retinopathy surrounding a choroidal melanoma treated with brachytherapy.** Marked lipid exudation is present at the necrotic tumor base.

LIPEMIA RETINALIS

Lipemia retinalis refers to salmon-colored retinal arteries and retinal veins due to elevated lipids, most commonly hypertriglyceridemia.

PATHOPHYSIOLOGY

- Elevated serum lipid levels may cause retinal vascular obstruction. The lipid abnormalities are typically heritable lipid metabolic abnormalities.

CLINICAL SIGNS

- Pale conjunctiva may result from lipemic conjunctival blood vessels. Fundus examination reveals salmon-colored retinal arteries and veins without skip areas (**Fig. 4-29**).

DIFFERENTIAL DIAGNOSIS

- Retinal vascular whitening can be observed in prior retinal vascular occlusion or in retinal vasculitis. These are typically confined to the retinal arterial or venous systems and typically have skip segments where the retinal vasculature is unaffected.

- Lipemia retinalis shows diffuse retinal arterial and venous involvement.

DIAGNOSTIC EVALUATION

- Fundus biomicroscopic examination reveals the characteristic retinal appearance described earlier and usually suffices to prompt systemic lipid evaluation.

- Fluorescein angiography may be obtained to evaluate retinal perfusion; areas of retinal telangiectasia may be observed.

- Family members should be evaluated, and systemic evaluation is indicated because of potential problems such as pancreatitis.

PROGNOSIS AND MANAGEMENT

- The visual prognosis can be good for patients who do not develop retinal vascular occlusive disease.

- Treatment is directed toward decreasing the causative lipemic factor.

FIGURE 4-29. **Lipemia retinalis. A.** A patient with markedly elevated triglyceride lipid levels who presented with a branch retinal vein occlusion and lipemic yellow retinal vessels and microaneurysms. **B.** After treatment with oral lipid-lowering agents, the retinal vasculature assumes normal coloring.

Retinal Degenerations and Dystrophies

Mithlesh C. Sharma and Allen C. Ho ■

BEST'S DISEASE

Best's disease, also known as vitelliform macular dystrophy, is a macular dystrophy that is clinically characterized by an egg yolk-like lesion at the level of the retinal pigment epithelium (RPE), usually located in the posterior pole. The disease progresses through various stages to culminate in macular atrophy or scarring with loss of central vision.

EPIDEMIOLOGY AND ETIOLOGY

- Symptoms develop in infancy or early childhood.

- An excessive amount of lipofuscin-like material within the retinal pigment epithelial cells, particularly in the fovea, is observed. There appears to be a secondary loss of the photoreceptor cells.

- It is an autosomal-dominant disease whose gene is mapped to chromosome 11q13.

CLINICAL SIGNS

- Five stages are delineated.

  1. Previtelliform stage: Patients are asymptomatic with no fundus abnormality, but electrooculography shows a reduced light-peak to dark-trough ratio.

  2. Vitelliform stage: This stage is characterized by an egg yolk-like lesion in the macular area. It is usually detected during the first or second decade of life. Although usually single and bilaterally symmetric, multiple egg yolk lesions may be observed in the posterior pole. The egg yolk lesions are located at the level of the RPE, are rounded or oval in shape with distinct borders, and range from one-half to two disc diameters in size. Vision may be normal or slightly decreased at this stage (Fig. 5-1).

  3. Pseudohypopyon stage: By the second or third decade of life, lesions break through the RPE, and the yellow material accumulates inferiorly in the macula

within the subretinal space to form pseudohypopyon (Fig. 5-2).

4. Vitelliruptive stage: The egg yolk breaks up to produce a scrambled egg appearance. Patients usually notice some visual impairment at this stage (Fig. 5-3).

5. End stage: Subretinal fibrosis, or a vascularized scar with choroidal neovascularization, contributes to the visual loss at this stage.

• The vitelliform degeneration presenting after childhood is called adult Best's disease. In the latter variant, the yellow foveal deposits are symmetric and similar to childhood Best's disease except that the lesions are smaller and have a central pigmented spot. The most common lesion mistaken for Best's disease is a yellow premacular hemorrhage (Fig. 5-4).

DIAGNOSTIC EVALUATION

• Visual acuity: Vision remains good while the egg yolk lesions are intact. Disruption or scarring of the lesions may reduce visual acuity to the level of 20/200.

• Visual fields: Central visual fields are normal initially, but a relative scotoma may develop with time.

• Color vision: Mild dyschromatopsia may be noticed.

• Dark adaptometry is normal.

• Electroretinography is normal.

• Electrooculography: Best's disease is one of the few conditions that results in an abnormal electrooculogram (EOG) in the setting of a normal electroretinogram (ERG). During an EOG, the light-peak:dark-trough ratio (Arden ratio) is typically below 1.5.

• Fluorescein angiography: In the vitelliform stage, complete blockage of background choroidal fluorescence by the lesion is observed. Areas of hyperfluorescence due to atrophic RPE are noticed as the egg yolk lesions show disruption.

PROGNOSIS AND MANAGEMENT

• In general, the overall prognosis is good as most patients retain reading level of vision in at least one eye throughout life.

• When severe vision loss does take place in an eye, it occurs slowly and usually begins after the age of 40 years.

• No treatment is available for Best's disease.

FIGURE 5-1. Best's disease, vitelliform stage. A. Characteristic egg yolk-like lesion in the fovea.
B. Corresponding fluorescein angiogram showing blocked fluorescence due to egg yolk lesion during transit phase. (Courtesy of Retina Slide Collection, Wills Eye Hospital, Philadelphia, Pennsylvania, compiled by Dr. Tamara Vrabec and Dr. Gordon Byrnes.)

FIGURE 5-2. **Best's disease, pseudohypopyon stage. A.** Collection of yellow material within the subretinal space simulating hypopyon (*arrow*). **B.** Blocked fluorescence (*arrow*) due to deposition of yellow material inferiorly and perifoveal hyperfluorescence in the center of the lesion is seen in fluorescein angiogram photographs. Courtesy of Retina Slide Collection, Wills Eye Hospital, Philadelphia, Pennsylvania, compiled by Dr. Tamara Vrabec and Dr. Gordon Byrnes.)

FIGURE 5-3. Best's disease, vitelliruptive stage. A. Irregular areas of retinal pigment epithelial loss secondary to breakup of the egg yolk lesion (*arrow*). **B.** Intense perifoveal hyperfluorescence surrounded by multiple areas of hyperfluorescence is shown in the corresponding fluorescein angiogram. (Courtesy of Retina Slide Collection, Wills Eye Hospital, Philadelphia, Pennsylvania, compiled by Dr. Tamara Vrabec and Dr. Gordon Byrnes.)

FIGURE 5-4. **Pseudo–Best's disease. A.** Old premacular hemorrhage simulating the egg yolk lesion of Best's disease. Note that the retinal vessels are obscured by the preretinal lesion (*arrow*). Slightly irregular borders of the lesion and presence of neighboring retinal hemorrhages are clues to the yellow lesion being an old hemorrhage. **B.** Fluorescein angiogram demonstrating microaneurysms and retinal telangiectasia temporal to the lesion, consistent with diabetic retinopathy and a premacular hemorrhage.

CONE DYSTROPHY

Cone dystrophy is an inherited defect that primarily affects the cone photoreceptor system.

EPIDEMIOLOGY AND ETIOLOGY

- Symptoms begin in early childhood to middle adulthood.
- Cone dystrophy is primarily autosomal dominant, although autosomal-recessive and X-linked forms have also been reported.

HISTORY

- The rate of progression and the severity of signs and symptoms are variable. The symptoms consist of progressive visual loss, hemeralopia (decreased vision in brightly illuminated environment), color vision difficulties, and central visual field defects.
- Macular changes typically follow the visual disturbances; therefore, early in the disease process the fundus may appear entirely normal.

CLINICAL SIGNS

- There is gradual, typically symmetric loss of visual acuity to the level of 20/200. Occasionally, this may be reduced to the level of counting fingers to hand motion acuity.
- Fundus changes are variable (Fig. 5-5). Early in the disease process, pigmentary stippling with diffuse pigment granularity in the posterior pole is the most common abnormality observed. The classic "bull's-eye" pattern of retinal pigment epithelial atrophy is a late finding. In advanced cases, a round, discrete area of central atrophy is seen. Temporal pallor of the optic disc may be observed.

DIFFERENTIAL DIAGNOSIS

- Reduced vision with normal fundus in children: In this category, cone dystrophy should be differentiated from Stargardt's disease.
- "Bull's-eye" maculopathy: The following causes of "bull's-eye" maculopathy need to be considered in the differential diagnosis:
  - Stargardt's disease
  - Chloroquine toxicity
  - Batten's disease
  - Benign concentric annular macular dystrophy
  - Leber's congenital amaurosis

DIAGNOSTIC EVALUATION

- Visual fields: Central scotoma is usually seen.
- Color vision: Reduced.
- Dark adaptometry: The cone component of the dark adaptation curve is abnormal.
- Electroretinography: The single-flash photopic ERG and the photopic flicker ERG are low or unrecordable. The scotopic ERG is usually normal.
- Fluorescein angiography: The retinal pigment epithelial changes in the macular area may be visible by fluorescein angiography before they can be visualized clinically. Early in the disease process, a mottled hyperfluorescence is seen. As the "bull's-eye" pattern of retinal pigment epithelial loss develops, hyperfluorescence surrounding a central area of hypofluorescence is observed.

PROGNOSIS AND MANAGEMENT

- The visual loss is gradual and symmetric to the level of 20/200. However, it may occasionally be severe enough to cause a visual acuity of counting fingers to hand motion. The visual loss is more severe in early-onset cases.
- No treatment is available for cone dystrophy.

FIGURE 5-5. Cone dystrophy. A. Early "bull's-eye" maculopathy in a patient with cone dystrophy (inset). Note the temporal optic disc atrophy (*arrow*). **B.** Corresponding fluorescein angiogram showing central hypofluorescence surrounded by a ring of hyperfluorescence seen during the transit phase (box).

(*continued*)

FIGURE 5-5. (*Continued*) **Cone dystrophy. C.** The hyperfluorescence fades away in the later frame indicating the presence of window defects due to retinal pigment epithelial atrophy. **D.** Advanced cone dystrophy with a classic "bull's-eye" maculopathy. Note the temporal optic disc pallor. (Courtesy of Dr. Joseph Maguire and the Retina Slide Collection, Wills Eye Hospital, Philadelphia, Pennsylvania, compiled by Dr. Tamara Vrabec and Dr. Gordon Byrnes.)

PATTERN DYSTROPHY

Pattern dystrophy describes a group of related conditions that are inherited in an autosomal-dominant fashion and are clinically characterized by variably shaped yellow or gray deposits in the macula.

EPIDEMIOLOGY AND ETIOLOGY

• Symptoms begin in middle age.

• The disease has an autosomal-dominant pattern. Genetic analysis of patients with butterfly dystrophy has shown mutation in the peripherin/RDS gene, located on the short arm of chromosome 6. The peripherin gene product plays an important role in the structural integrity of photoreceptor outer segment discs. However, this mutation does not correspond to a particular phenotype. That is, other forms of retinal degeneration have been linked to peripherin/RDS gene mutations.

HISTORY

• Most patients are either asymptomatic or have minimal visual disturbances. Typically, the diagnosis is made on routine fundus examination of a middle-aged adult.

CLINICAL SIGNS

• Visual acuity: Patients may have normal visual acuity up to the fifth or sixth decade of life. Reduced vision and metamorphopsia may be the presenting symptoms.

• Ophthalmoscopically: The following patterns of pigment deposits in the macular area may be observed:

■ Most commonly, a bilateral, triradiate ("butterfly") pattern of yellow or gray pigment at the level of the RPE in the central

macular region. A rim of retinal pigment epithelial atrophy around the pigment figure, which is more apparent on fluorescein angiography, may also be seen (**Figs. 5-6 and 5-7**).

■ A single, round, vitelliform lesion in the fovea (adult-onset foveomacular vitelliform dystrophy).

■ Extensive macular fishnet arrangement (reticular dystrophy).

■ Coarse pigment mottling of the macula (fundus pulverulentus) (**Fig. 5-8**).

• The affected members of a given pedigree may have different patterns, and the patterns may differ in the eyes of an affected individual. Even a change from one to another pattern over time may be observed.

DIFFERENTIAL DIAGNOSIS

• Large drusen: Ophthalmoscopically, the yellow pigment figures of pattern dystrophy may be confused with the large drusen of age-related macular degeneration.

DIAGNOSTIC EVALUATION

• Visual fields: Normal, except for minimally reduced sensitivity in the macular area.

• Color vision, dark adaptometry, electroretinography: Normal.

• Electrooculography: Mildly abnormal, which is consistent with the disturbed retinal pigment epithelial function.

• Fluorescein angiography: Pigment figures are hypofluorescent throughout the study. The retinal pigment epithelial atrophy around the lesions produces hyperfluorescence.

PROGNOSIS

• The prognosis for retention of good central vision in at least one eye throughout life is excellent.

FIGURE 5-6. Pattern dystrophy. A and **B.** Bilateral, multiple, discrete, yellow areas at the level of the retinal pigment epithelium (RPE) in the central macular region (inset).

(*continued*)

FIGURE 5-6. (*Continued*) **Pattern dystrophy. C.** The lesions are more pronounced in the corresponding fluorescein angiogram image of the right eye, where there is patchy hyperfluorescence.

FIGURE 5-7. Pattern dystrophy. A. Classic triradiate ("butterfly") pattern of pigment deposits at the fovea (inset) surrounded by multiple areas of retinal pigment epithelial atrophy. **B.** Fluorescein angiogram showing patchy hyperfluorescence in the arteriovenous phase. The hyperfluorescent areas correspond to retinal pigment epithelial atrophy in the macular region. (Courtesy of Dr. Eric Shakin and the Retina Slide Collection, Wills Eye Hospital, Philadelphia, Pennsylvania, compiled by Dr. Tamara Vrabec and Dr. Gordon Byrnes.)

FIGURE 5-8. Pattern dystrophy, fundus pulverulentus. Fluorescein angiogram photographs of both eyes showing radiating pattern of hypofluorescence due to coarse pigment deposits at the level of RPE—reticular dystrophy. (Courtesy of Dr. William Annesley, and the Retina Slide Collection, Wills Eye Hospital, Philadelphia, Pennsylvania, compiled by Dr. Tamara Vrabec and Dr. Gordon Byrnes.)

STARGARDT'S DISEASE

Stargardt's disease is a macular dystrophy that is characterized by the presence of discrete, yellow, pisciform flecks at the level of the RPE. Currently, Stargardt's disease and fundus flavimaculatus are regarded as variants of the same disorder. The term *fundus flavimaculatus* is generally applied when the characteristic flecks are scattered throughout the fundus. When the flecks are confined to the posterior pole and are associated with macular atrophy, the condition is described as Stargardt's disease.

EPIDEMIOLOGY AND ETIOLOGY

- The disease usually presents in the first or second decade of life.
- Both sexes are affected equally.
- Stargardt's disease is usually autosomal recessive, although dominantly inherited cases have been described. The gene for autosomal-recessive Stargardt's disease is located on chromosome 1. This gene codes for an ATP-binding transport protein (ABCR) that is expressed in the rod inner segments, but not the RPE. A homozygous mutation in the ABCR gene causes fundus flavimaculatus.

HISTORY

- Children with Stargardt's disease are usually brought to the attention of an ophthalmologist as a result of a gradual impairment of vision noticed by the parents or after failing a school vision screening.

CLINICAL SIGNS

- Visual acuity is slightly affected in the beginning but may be severely reduced in the later stage of disease. Loss of the foveal reflex may be the only initial clinical finding. Discrete, yellowish, "pisciform" flecks located at the level of the RPE are often noticed at some point in the course of disease. The flecks may or may not involve the macula (Fig. 5-9). Perifoveal retinal pigment epithelial mottling may become evident with the progression of disease.
- A "bull's-eye" pattern of retinal pigment epithelial loss may become apparent, particularly by fluorescein angiography. The macula classically develops a "beaten bronze" appearance corresponding to atrophy of the central RPE in the advanced stage of disease (Figs. 5-10 and 5-11). Histopathology shows an accumulation of an abnormal lipofuscin-like material in the RPE (Fig. 5-12).

DIFFERENTIAL DIAGNOSIS

- Cone dystrophy: reduced vision and normal fundus in a child
- "Bull's-eye" maculopathy: chloroquine toxicity, Batten's disease, benign concentric annular macular dystrophy

DIAGNOSTIC EVALUATION

- Visual fields: Usually a central scotoma is noted, but a paracentral scotoma, central constriction, and a ring scotoma may also be seen, especially early in the disease.
- Color vision: Mild dyschromatopsia to red and green may be noted.
- Dark adaptometry: Dark adaptation may be delayed.
- Fluorescein angiography: Features that may help confirm the diagnosis of Stargardt's disease include dark or silent choroid;

multiple, irregular hyperfluorescent spots that do not precisely correspond to the flecks; and a "bull's-eye" window-defect pattern of hyperfluorescence in the macula.

- Electroretinography: Usually normal but may be reduced with increasing amounts of peripheral flecks and atrophy.

- Electrooculography: Usually subnormal.

PROGNOSIS AND MANAGEMENT

- The majority of patients preserve moderate visual acuity (20/70 to 20/200), at least in one eye.

- No effective treatment is available for Stargardt's disease.

FIGURE 5-9. Stargardt's disease. A. Multiple, discrete, yellow, "pisciform" flecks (inset shows one fleck) located at the level of the RPE with corresponding hyperfluorescent areas in the fluorescein angiogram photograph are distributed throughout the posterior pole of the left eye. **B.** The background choroid is dark on the fluorescein angiogram photograph, and there is transmission hyperfluorescence associated with macular flecks and retinal pigment epithelial alterations. (Courtesy of Retina Slide Collection, Wills Eye Hospital, Philadelphia, Pennsylvania, compiled by Dr. Tamara Vrabec and Dr. Gordon Byrnes.)

FIGURE 5-10. Stargardt's disease. A. Advanced Stargardt's disease with "beaten bronze" macula.
B. Corresponding fluorescein angiogram showing a central area of hypofluorescence (retinal pigment epithelial clumping) surrounded by a ring of hyperfluorescence (retinal pigment epithelial atrophy). Note the dark or silent choroid (blocked fluorescence).

(continued)

C

FIGURE 5-10. (*Continued*) **Stargardt's disease. C.** Stargardt's disease with "bull's-eye" macula. Compare with Figure 5-5D. Note the "beaten bronze" appearance of the macula (inset). (Courtesy of Dr. Eric Shakin and the Retina Slide Collection, Wills Eye Hospital, Philadelphia, Pennsylvania, compiled by Dr. Tamara Vrabec and Dr. Gordon Byrnes.)

FIGURE 5-11. **Stargardt's disease. A.** Severe loss of RPE in a geographic fashion in the central macular region in a patient with advanced Stargardt's disease. The visual acuity was reduced to 20/200. **B.** Corresponding fluorescein angiogram showing irregularly distributed areas of hypofluorescence and hyperfluorescence, with a discrete rim of hyperfluorescence within the area of geographic pattern of retinal pigment epithelial loss. Dark choroid is apparent beyond the macula.

FIGURE 5-12. **Stargardt's disease, electron microphotograph.** Electron microphotograph showing enlarged retinal pigment epithelial cells due to intracellular accumulation of lipofuscin-like material. (Courtesy of Dr. Ralph Eagle, Wills Eye Hospital, Philadelphia, Pennsylvania.)

CHOROIDEREMIA

Choroideremia is a generalized hereditary retinal degeneration that primarily affects the choriocapillaris and the RPE–photoreceptor complex.

EPIDEMIOLOGY AND ETIOLOGY

- Symptoms are usually noted in the first or second decade of life.
- Only males are affected, and females are carriers.
- Choroideremia is an X-linked recessive disorder.

HISTORY

- Patients usually present in the first or second decade of life with a chief complaint of difficulty with night vision.

CLINICAL SIGNS

- Early in the disease process, fundus appearance in the affected males is a "salt-and-pepper" retinal pigment epithelial mottling at the equator and the posterior pole. Below the retinal pigment epithelial mottling, the underlying choroid may appear clinically normal, but fluorescein angiography may show a patchy loss of choroidal vasculature.
- Later in the disease process, small areas of the RPE drop out in the midperiphery. These areas of drop-out eventually coalesce and progress centrally. The macula is involved last (Fig. 5-13). In the final stages, the entire fundus, with an exception of the macula, shows the diffuse yellow–white reflex of the underlying sclera.
- Female carriers show unique and pathognomonic fundus features. The generalized retinal pigment epithelial mottling, especially in the midperiphery, resembles the changes seen in males in the early stage of disease. The fundus changes in female carriers remain stationary, and the fluorescein angiography reveals an intact choroidal vasculature.

DIFFERENTIAL DIAGNOSIS

- Retinitis pigmentosa: Unlike retinitis pigmentosa (RP), in choroideremia a "bone-spicule" pattern of pigmentary change is usually not seen, and the retinal blood vessels remain relatively normal.
- Gyrate atrophy: In the final stages, fundus appearance in choroideremia may resemble gyrate atrophy, but the different mode of genetic transmission is an important distinguishing feature.

DIAGNOSTIC EVALUATION

- Visual Fields: There is a loss of peripheral visual field.
- Electroretinography: This may be normal during the early stage, but by the end of the first decade the scotopic ERG becomes nonrecordable and the photopic ERG is severely reduced.
- Fluorescein angiography: In the early stage, despite the clinically normal-appearing choroid, fluorescein angiography may reveal a patchy loss of choriocapillaris. Later in the disease, an extensive loss of choroidal vasculature is observed (Figs. 5-14 and 5-15).

PROGNOSIS AND MANAGEMENT

• Relatively good central vision is preserved until late in the disease because the macula is affected late. Although the rate of progression may vary within a pedigree, the majority of patients usually have severely reduced vision by the age of 35 years.

• Female carriers usually retain normal visual function throughout their life.

• No treatment is available for choroideremia.

FIGURE 5-13. Choroideremia. Multiple areas of retinal pigment epithelial loss, some of which have coalesced to form larger patches. Note that the fovea is spared and the patient had 20/40 vision in this eye. (Courtesy of Retina Slide Collection, Wills Eye Hospital, Philadelphia, Pennsylvania, compiled by Dr. Tamara Vrabec and Dr. Gordon Byrnes.)

FIGURE 5-14. Early choroideremia. Peripapillary loss of the RPE (**A**) and subtle pigmentary mottling in the midperipheral fundus (**B**) can be seen (inset). Similar fundus findings can be observed in female carriers of choroideremia. (Courtesy of Retina Slide Collection, Wills Eye Hospital, Philadelphia, Pennsylvania, compiled by Dr. Tamara Vrabec and Dr. Gordon Byrnes.)

FIGURE 5-15. Late choroideremia. A. Extensive loss of choriocapillaris is evident in the corresponding late-phase fluorescein angiogram photograph (same patient as in Figure 5-13A). **B.** Equator-plus red-free fundus photograph showing multiple patches of the retinal pigment epithelial loss extending from the posterior pole to the midperiphery (same patient as in Figure 5-13B). (Courtesy of Retina Slide Collection, Wills Eye Hospital, Philadelphia, Pennsylvania, compiled by Dr. Tamara Vrabec and Dr. Gordon Byrnes.)

GYRATE ATROPHY

Gyrate atrophy is a rare choroidal disorder, which is usually transmitted in an autosomal-recessive fashion and is caused by an absence or near-absence of the pyridoxine-dependent mitochondrial matrix enzyme ornithine aminotransferase.

EPIDEMIOLOGY AND ETIOLOGY

- Symptoms begin in the first decade of life.
- The disorder is autosomal recessive.
- Elevated levels of ornithine in the plasma and urine in patients with gyrate atrophy are caused by an absence or near-absence of the pyridoxine-dependent mitochondrial matrix enzyme ornithine aminotransferase. The latter is necessary for the breakdown of excess ornithine in humans.

HISTORY

- The usual presenting symptoms are poor night vision and constricted visual fields.

CLINICAL SIGNS

- Early in the disease, a thinning and transparency of the RPE, beginning in the midperiphery, is observed. The underlying choroid may appear either normal or sclerotic. The affected areas are separated from the normal-appearing retina by scalloped borders. The involved areas begin as isolated patches but later coalesce (**Fig. 5-16**).
- Progression of the disease is accompanied by pigment clumping and choroidal atrophy. Eventually the entire choroidal vasculature disappears, exposing the white sclera. The optic disc and the retinal vessels may be normal early in the disease, as time passes blood vessels show a gradual narrowing.
- In the later stages, marked choroidal atrophy from the periphery to the posterior pole is evident. However, the macula is usually spared. Macular involvement may be in the form of macular edema or related to progression of atrophic changes.

ASSOCIATED CLINICAL SIGNS

- Ocular
  - Myopia: Almost invariably present
  - Cataract: Seen in a high proportion of patients with gyrate atrophy
- Systemic
  - Characteristically thin, sparse, straight hair
  - Less consistent findings: Abnormal electroencephalogram, muscle weakness, abnormal electrocardiogram, and seizures

DIFFERENTIAL DIAGNOSIS

- Choroideremia: In late stages, fundus appearance of choroideremia and gyrate atrophy can be remarkably similar. However, different modes of genetic transmission and the distinctive fundus features in the female carriers of choroideremia are important distinguishing features.

DIAGNOSTIC EVALUATION

- Visual fields: Constriction of the peripheral visual fields corresponds to the expansion of the fundus changes.
- Fluorescein angiography: A loss of choriocapillaris is demonstrated in the affected areas.
- Electroretinography: Severely diminished or abolished amplitudes.

- Electrooculography: Abnormal.

- Other: Elevated serum ornithine levels and markedly decreased ornithine aminotransferase activity in cultured fibroblasts or leukocytes.

PROGNOSIS AND MANAGEMENT

- Patients are usually legally blind by the fourth to seventh decade of life. However, earlier visual loss may result from cataract.

- Pyridoxine (vitamin B6) may help normalize the plasma and urinary ornithine levels and preserve visual function. On the basis of a response to vitamin B6, gyrate atrophy may have two clinically different subtypes. Patients responsive to vitamin B6 usually have a less severe and more slowly progressive clinical course than patients who are not responsive.

- A low-protein diet, particularly a low-arginine diet, may also be of benefit.

FIGURE 5-16. **Gyrate atrophy. A.** Bilateral, multiple, geographic patches of retinal pigment epithelial loss with scalloped borders (inset) are present in the posterior pole and the peripapillary area. **B.** Scattered pigmentary clumping is also visible.

(*continued*)

FIGURE 5-16. (*Continued*) **Gyrate atrophy. C** and **D.** Extensive atrophy of the RPE and the choroidal vasculature is evident in the corresponding fluorescein angiogram photographs. The fovea is spared in both eyes, and the patient's visual acuity was 20/40 OD, 20/30 OS. (Courtesy of Retina Slide Collection, Wills Eye Hospital, Philadelphia, Pennsylvania, compiled by Dr. Tamara Vrabec and Dr. Gordon Byrnes.)

CONGENITAL STATIONARY NIGHT BLINDNESS

Congenital stationary night blindness (CSNB) is a group of disorders that is characterized by defective night vision, which remains stable throughout life.

CLASSIFICATION

● CSNB with normal fundus appearance.
● CSNB with abnormal fundus appearance: This group includes fundus albipunctatus and Oguchi's disease.

FUNDUS ALBIPUNCTATUS

Fundus albipunctatus (FA) is a disorder of the visual pigment regeneration process that is characterized by an abnormally prolonged recovery of normal rhodopsin levels following an intense light exposure.

HISTORY

● The presenting symptom is nonprogressive impaired night vision, but given enough time to adapt in the dark, patients will achieve a normal sensitivity.

EPIDEMIOLOGY AND ETIOLOGY

● The proposed defect in patients with FA appears to be an abnormal regeneration rate of the visual photoreceptor pigments.
● Autosomal recessive.

CLINICAL SIGNS

● Visual acuity: Usually unaffected.
● Fundus: Examination shows a multitude of yellow–white, tiny dots in the posterior pole that radiate out toward the periphery. The macula is almost invariably spared (Fig. 5-17).

DIFFERENTIAL DIAGNOSIS

● Retinitis punctata albescens: This is a variant of RP in which the fundus shows yellow–white dots but has narrowed vessels and a severely reduced ERG that does not recover with dark adaptation.
● Fleck retina of Kandori: A disorder with larger patch-like flecks and a less severe impairment of night vision.

DIAGNOSTIC EVALUATION

● Visual fields: Normal.
● Dark adaptometry: Both the cone and rod components of the dark adaptation curve are very slow in reaching the final threshold.
● Electroretinography: It is important to know that unless given enough time to dark adapt, both the a- and b-waves of the ERG are severely reduced. However, with prolonged dark adaptation, ERG returns to normal.
● Electrooculography: There is a slow recovery of the light rise with dark adaptation.

PROGNOSIS AND MANAGEMENT

● The defective night vision is nonprogressive, and the vision is usually unaffected.

FIGURE 5-17. Fundus albipunctatus. Multiple tiny yellow–white dots radiating out from the posterior pole toward the fundus periphery.

OGUCHI'S DISEASE

O guchi's disease is a variant of CSNB characterized by a nonprogressive night vision impairment that is thought to be due to a defective phototransduction process.

EPIDEMIOLOGY AND ETIOLOGY

- The visual photoreceptor pigments are normal, and the proposed defect is thought to be impaired phototransduction, giving rise to abnormal ERG findings.

CLINICAL SIGNS

- The retina has a peculiar silvery metallic sheen where retinal vessels stand out against the background fundus appearance. This unusual appearance may be seen in the entire retina or may be present only in the posterior pole or the periphery.
- **Mizuo–Nakamura phenomenon:** The retina has a metallic sheen following light adaptation, which disappears after few hours in the dark (Fig. 5-18).

DIAGNOSTIC EVALUATION

- Visual fields: Normal.
- Dark adaptometry: There is a normal cone adaptation but a markedly delayed rod adaptation that reaches a normal threshold level over a prolonged period of time (from 3 to 24 hours).
- Electroretinography: Normal-amplitude a-wave and reduced or absent b-wave are seen under photopic and scotopic conditions. It is of note that even after the dark-adapted thresholds have returned to normal, the ERG b-wave may still be absent.
- Electrooculography: Normal light rise.

PROGNOSIS AND MANAGEMENT

- The night vision defect is nonprogressive.
- There is no treatment available for Oguchi's disease.

FIGURE 5-18. Mizuo–Nakamura phenomenon. Metallic sheen of the retina after light exposure (right-hand photographs) has disappeared after a few hours of dark adaptation (left). (Courtesy of Retina Slide Collection, Wills Eye Hospital, Philadelphia, Pennsylvania, compiled by Dr. Tamara Vrabec and Dr. Gordon Byrnes.)

ALBINISM

Albinism is a group of conditions that involves the melanin system of the eye or skin, or both.

CLASSIFICATION

- Ophthalmically, two clinical patterns are noted:
  - True albinism: Congenitally subnormal vision and nystagmus are present.
  - Albinoidism: There is normal or minimally reduced vision and no nystagmus.
- However, both clinical patterns share many clinical characteristics. True albinism is divided into the following two types:
  - Oculocutaneous albinism: Both the eye and the skin are affected.
  - Ocular albinism: Only the eyes appear to be affected.

EPIDEMIOLOGY AND ETIOLOGY

- Oculocutaneous albinism results from a reduction in the amount of primary melanin deposited in each melanosome, whereas ocular albinism is caused by a reduction in the total number of melanosomes.
- Genetics
  - Oculocutaneous albinism: autosomal recessive
  - Ocular albinism: X-linked

IMPORTANT CLINICAL SIGNS

- Both ocular and oculocutaneous albinism share the following ocular clinical features:
  - Reduced visual acuity in the range of 20/40 to 20/400. The severity of visual deficit is proportional to the degree of fundus hypopigmentation (Fig. 5-19).
  - Nystagmus, light sensitivity, and a high degree of refractive errors.
  - Iris transillumination from decreased pigmentation.
  - Foveal aplasia or hypoplasia. In the presence of significant foveal hypoplasia, nystagmus begins within 2 to 3 months of life (Fig. 5-20).
  - Hypopigmented retina from the periphery to the posterior pole.
  - Abnormal retinogeniculostriate projections where many temporal nerve fibers decussate rather than project to the ipsilateral geniculate body. This phenomenon accounts for the abnormal stereopsis in these patients.
- The female carriers of ocular albinism may reveal partial iris transillumination and fundus hypopigmentation (Fig. 5-21).

ASSOCIATED CLINICAL SIGNS

- Skin hypopigmentation is seen in patients with oculocutaneous albinism. Two forms of potentially lethal albinisms are observed:
  - Chédiak–Higashi syndrome: Oculocutaneous albinism is combined with extreme susceptibility to infection that can often lead to death in childhood or youth.
  - Hermansky–Pudlak syndrome: Oculocutaneous albinism with a platelet defect causing easy bruising and bleeding. Most patients with this disorder in the United States are of Puerto Rican origin.

HISTOLOGY

- Macromelanosomes in the eye or skin, or both

- Increased number of decussating fibers at the chiasm

DIAGNOSTIC EVALUATION

- The typical constellation of symptoms and signs suggests the diagnosis. Asymmetric visually evoked cortical potentials occur due to abnormal decussation of the nerve fibers at the chiasm.

- The tyrosinase hair bulb test indicates the presence or absence of the tyrosinase enzyme (it is required in the biosynthesis of melanin) and divides the oculocutaneous albinism into two types, tyrosinase-positive and tyrosinase-negative. Tyrosinase-negative albinos show a complete lack of pigmentation in the skin, hair, and eyes, whereas tyrosinase-positive albinos have some degree of pigmentation.

- Hematologic consultation is necessary if Chédiak–Higashi or Hermansky–Pudlak syndromes are suspected (**Fig. 5-22**).

PROGNOSIS AND MANAGEMENT

- Since all forms of albinism are inherited, genetic counseling is important. A majority of children with albinism are able to attend regular schools with some degree of assistance, but only a few see well enough to drive.

- Refraction, tinted glasses, and visual aids are helpful for older patients.

- Hematologic consultation in an appropriate setting is mandatory.

FIGURE 5-19. Albinism. Markedly hypopigmented fundus. Note the haphazard underlying large choroidal vessels. (Courtesy of Retina Slide Collection, Wills Eye Hospital, Philadelphia, Pennsylvania, compiled by Dr. Tamara Vrabec and Dr. Gordon Byrnes.)

FIGURE 5-20. **Albinism, foveal hypoplasia.** Color fundus photograph concentrating on the foveal region of a patient with albinism. Note a complete absence of foveal architecture and foveal reflex—foveal hypoplasia (box). (Courtesy of Retina Slide Collection, Wills Eye Hospital, Philadelphia, Pennsylvania, compiled by Dr. Tamara Vrabec and Dr. Gordon Byrnes.)

FIGURE 5-21. **Albinism, female carrier.** Partially hypopigmented fundus in a female carrier of ocular albinism. (Courtesy of Retina Slide Collection, Wills Eye Hospital, Philadelphia, Pennsylvania, compiled by Dr. Tamara Vrabec and Dr. Gordon Byrnes.)

FIGURE 5-22. **Oculocutaneous albinism, Hermansky–Pudlak Syndrome.** Purpuric patches on the cheeks, forehead, and left upper lid of a young boy with oculocutaneous albinism and Hermansky–Pudlak syndrome. (Courtesy of Retina Slide Collection, Wills Eye Hospital, Philadelphia, Pennsylvania, compiled by Dr. Tamara Vrabec and Dr. Gordon Byrnes.)

RETINITIS PIGMENTOSA

RP is a group of hereditary disorders associated with a primary abnormality of the photoreceptor–RPE complex, and is characterized subjectively by night blindness and a loss of peripheral vision, and objectively by a grossly reduced or extinguished full-field ERG. However, the hereditary basis can be established in only 50% of cases.

EPIDEMIOLOGY AND ETIOLOGY

- Onset: Variable and depends on the inheritance pattern.
- Genetics: The following modes of inheritance have been described:
  - Sporadic: There is no family history of RP. These are the most common cases. Some of these cases are autosomal recessive, and others may represent autosomal-dominant mutations.
  - Autosomal dominant: The next most common mode of inheritance and has the best prognosis.
  - Autosomal recessive.
  - X-linked recessive: Least common group with worst prognosis.

HISTORY

- Patients with typical RP present with a history of night blindness or nyctalopia (a complete or partially reduced rate of visual adaptation at night or in dim illumination). Patients may also have difficulty with peripheral vision in dim light.
- The difficulty with night vision may begin in early childhood, or patients may notice it in the second or third decade of life. By the age of 30 years, over 75% of patients are symptomatic.

CLINICAL SIGNS

- The classic clinical triad of RP includes (Fig. 5-23):
  - Retinal "bone-spicule" pigmentation
  - Arteriolar attenuation
  - Waxy optic disc pallor (Fig. 5-24)
- Additionally, vitreous debris is frequently encountered.

Important Clinical Signs

- Night blindness: The most common presenting clinical symptom. Peripheral vision problems are initially noticed only in the dim light, but later these problems are noted under all conditions. Eventually, only a small zone of central vision remains.
- Visual acuity: The central vision may be preserved for many years in the autosomal-dominant form of RP. An early loss of central vision is often observed in the X-linked or autosomal-recessive forms. Additionally, cataract, cystoid macular edema, and surface wrinkling of the internal limiting membrane may contribute to early vision loss.
- Fundus findings: Fundus findings may differ according to the stage of the disease.
  - Very early: Arteriolar narrowing; fine dust-like intraretinal pigmentation.
  - Later features: Perivascular "bone-spicule" pigment clumping. Pigmentary changes begin in the midretinal periphery and then extend anteriorly as well as posteriorly, giving rise to a ring scotoma. Waxy pallor of the optic disc is the least reliable sign of the RP triad.
  - Advanced features: Unmasking of the large choroidal vessels, prominent arteriolar attenuation, and marked optic disc pallor.
- Macula: Macular involvement may occur in the following ways:

- Cystoid macular edema (may respond to systemic acetazolamide)
- Surface wrinkling
- Atrophic changes

Associated Ocular Features

- Optic nerve head drusen
- Open-angle glaucoma (in 3% of patients with RP)
- Posterior subcapsular cataract (common in all forms of RP)
- Keratoconus
- Myopia (frequently encountered)

DIAGNOSTIC EVALUATION

- A constellation of characteristic signs and symptoms helps establish the diagnosis.
- Visual fields: Initially, there is a full or partial ring scotoma in the midperiphery, which extends anteriorly as well as posteriorly, leaving only a central island of vision in the late stages.
- Dark adaptometry: An elevation of the rod as well as the cone segment of the dark adaptation curve occurs. On the basis of the dark adaptometry results, autosomal-dominant RP can be divided into two types:

    - Type I RP: Early-onset nyctalopia with an early diffuse loss of the rod sensitivity relative to cone sensitivity
    - Type II RP: Adult-onset nyctalopia with an equal loss of the rod and cone sensitivity

- Electroretinography: This may be significantly subnormal even when the fundus shows minimal changes. Severely reduced or almost extinguished scotopic ERG responses are observed, whereas the photopic ERG is relatively unaffected. The cone b-wave implicit times, as elicited by flicker stimuli, are almost always prolonged in all forms of electroretinography. The b-wave implicit time on the ERG may be prolonged in patients with predominant loss of rods rather than cones. Recently, distinctive ERG patterns in the type I and the type II autosomal-dominant forms of RP have been observed. The rod ERG is more severely affected than the cone ERG in type I RP, whereas rod and cone ERGs are equally abnormal in type II RP.

- Electrooculography: Almost invariably reduced.
- Atypical RP

    - Retinitis punctata albescens: Scattered white dots are located mostly between the posterior pole and the equator.
    - Sector RP: Only one or two quadrants of the fundus are involved (**Fig. 5-25**).
    - Pericentric RP: Pigmentary changes are confined to the area around the posterior pole.
    - RP sine pigmento: Pigmentary changes in the fundus are either minimal or absent.
    - RP with exudative vasculopathy: Coats' disease-like appearance in the fundus.

PROGNOSIS AND MANAGEMENT

- About one quarter of patients maintain good vision and are able to read throughout their lives. The autosomal-dominant form of the disease has the best prognosis, and the X-linked form has the worst prognosis.
- Only a few patients younger than 20 years of age have a visual acuity of 20/400 or less. By the age of 50 years, however, a significant proportion of patients will have a visual acuity of approximately 20/400.
- Electroretinography is helpful in identifying the female carriers of X-linked RP (who

may have a normal fundus), which may have implications for genetic counseling.

• Appropriate investigations should be performed to rule out atypical forms of RP that may have an associated treatable systemic condition. Explain to patients that not all people with RP go completely blind.

• Yearly follow-up is recommended to detect a precipitous fall in vision that may raise a possibility of a treatable cause, such as cystoid macular edema or cataract. Cystoid macular edema associated with RP responds favorably to oral acetazolamide, which is initially tried

in a dose of 125 mg twice a day for 2 months to confirm its beneficial effect. If effective, acetazolamide may need to be continued for many months in some patients.

• Serial Goldmann perimetry should be performed at regular intervals to assess visual field changes.

• The role of oral vitamin A therapy in slowing the rate of progression of typical RP remains controversial.

• A variety of low-vision aids may be helpful.

FIGURE 5-23. Retinitis pigmentosa (RP). The classic clinical triad of waxy optic disc pallor, arteriolar attenuation, and "bone-spicule" pigmentation (inset) in a patient with RP. (Courtesy of Retina Slide Collection, Wills Eye Hospital, Philadelphia, Pennsylvania, compiled by Dr. Tamara Vrabec and Dr. Gordon Byrnes.)

FIGURE 5-24. **RP.** Arteriolar attenuation (inset, **A**), optic disc pallor (arrow, **B**), and pigmentary changes in the fundus are the characteristic findings in patients with RP. Visual acuity was reduced to finger counting vision due to foveal changes. (Courtesy of Retina Slide Collection, Wills Eye Hospital, Philadelphia, Pennsylvania, compiled by Dr. Tamara Vrabec and Dr. Gordon Byrnes.)

FIGURE 5-25. RP, sector variant. Equator-plus color fundus photograph showing inferior sectorial retinal pigmentary changes. (Courtesy of Retina Slide Collection, Wills Eye Hospital, Philadelphia, Pennsylvania, compiled by Dr. Tamara Vrabec and Dr. Gordon Byrnes.)

SYSTEMIC DISEASES ASSOCIATED WITH RETINITIS PIGMENTOSA

USHER'S SYNDROME

Usher's syndrome is defined as congenital or progressive hearing loss associated with RP and is the most common syndrome associated with RP. Approximately 4% of children attending schools for the deaf have RP, and 50% of blind–deaf individuals have Usher's syndrome.

- Pigmentary retinopathy: It is progressive and develops before puberty.

- Systemic features: Usher's syndrome is divided into four subtypes, and types I and II constitute the majority of cases.

  - Type I: Profound congenital deafness, abnormal vestibular functions, and early-onset RP

  - Type II: Partial deafness, intact vestibular functions, and a milder form of RP

BASSEN–KORNZWEIG SYNDROME (ABETALIPOPROTEINEMIA)

This disorder is thought to be caused by an inability of the body to synthesize apolipoprotein B, which helps in the absorption of fats in the small intestine.

- Pigmentary retinopathy: It develops at the end of the first decade of life. Ptosis and ocular motility disturbances may also be seen.

- Systemic features: Spinocerebellar ataxia, acanthocytosis, and abetalipoproteinemia are noted. Fat malabsorption and associated deficiency of fat-soluble vitamins, particularly A and E, is present, and jejunal biopsy is diagnostic.

- Treatment: Supplementation of vitamins A and E may be beneficial. Oral supplementation of vitamin A to reverse the psychophysical and electrophysiologic abnormalities remains controversial.

REFSUM'S DISEASE (HEREDOPATHIA ATACTICA POLYNEURITIFORMIS)

Refsum's disease is an autosomal-recessive disorder caused by a metabolic abnormality that results in a deposition of phytanic acid in many body tissues, including the eyes.

- Pigmentary retinopathy: Nyctalopia is almost always present. Fundus pigmentation is generally of a "salt-and-pepper" rather than "bone-spicule" type.

- Systemic features: Hypertrophic peripheral neuropathy, cerebellar ataxia, deafness, ichthyosis, cardiac arrhythmias, and elevated cerebrospinal fluid protein.

- Treatment: Normalization of the elevated serum phytanic acid levels by a low phytanic acid diet may improve retinal function, and stop or slow the progression of disease.

COCKAYNE'S SYNDROME

- Pigmentary retinopathy: "Salt-and-pepper type" with arteriolar attenuation and optic nerve pallor.

- Systemic features: Childhood dwarfism with cachectic and prematurely aged appearance. Affected children have a small head with characteristic bird-like facies, and disproportionately large hands and feet. Deafness, photodermatitis, nystagmus, ataxia, and progressive mental retardation are associated features. Death may occur in the third or fourth decade of life.

KEARNS–SAYRE SYNDROME

This syndrome is a mitochondrial myopathy in which an increased number of distorted mitochondria are accumulated in the skeletal muscles (including the extraocular muscles), RPE, and heart. Histologically, affected muscles show "ragged-red" fibers, caused by the accumulation of mitochondria beneath the plasma membrane and between myofibrils.

● Pigmentary retinopathy: Variable appearance. Diffuse retinal pigment epithelial mottling may be observed.

● Systemic features: Combination of chronic progressive external ophthalmoplegia (most common finding), pigmentary retinopathy, and complete heart block (may cause death). This condition usually becomes manifest before the age of 20 years.

BARDET–BIEDL SYNDROME

● Pigmentary retinopathy: "Bull's-eye" maculopathy occurs in most cases. A few cases are similar to typical RP with "bone-spicule" pigmentation.

● Systemic features: Mental handicap, polydactyly, obesity, and hypogenitalism; renal abnormalities (in most cases).

LAURENCE–MOON SYNDROME

● Retinopathy: Either typical RP type or choroidal atrophy.

● Systemic features: Spastic paraplegia, mental handicap, and hypogenitalism.

MUCOPOLYSACCHARIDOSES

This group of metabolic disorders is caused by a deficiency of lysosomal enzymes involved in the degradation of many mucopolysaccharides, such as dermatan sulfate, heparan sulfate, and keratan sulfate. An abnormal deposition of the nondegraded mucopolysaccharides leads to multiple organ system dysfunction.

● Genetics: Autosomal recessive, except Hunter's disease, which is X-linked recessive.

● Ocular features: Retinal pigmentary degeneration—found in Hurler's, Hunter's, and Sanfilippo's diseases; corneal stromal infiltration; optic nerve head swelling; optic atrophy; and glaucoma (rare).

● Systemic features: Facial coarseness, skeletal anomalies, and heart disease.

NEURONAL CEROID LIPOFUSCINOSIS (BATTEN DISEASE)

This group of disorders is characterized by an accumulation of autofluorescent lipopigments in the neurons as well as in nonneural tissues. Four types are differentiated, as follows:

● Infantile type (Hagberg–Santavuori)

  ▪ Generalized retinal degeneration

  ▪ Brownish discoloration of the macula

  ▪ Early visual loss

  ▪ Optic atrophy

  ▪ Mental retardation and motor abnormalities between the ages of 1 and 1½ years

● Late infantile type (Jansky–Bielschowsky)

- Generalized retinal degeneration and optic atrophy

- Seizures and psychomotor problems with an onset between 2 and 4 years of age

- Juvenile type (Spielmeyer–Vogt)
  - Most common
  - "Bull's-eye" maculopathy with eventual development of RP-like clinical picture: May need to be differentiated from Stargardt's disease
  - Reduced vision
  - Progressive mental deterioration
  - Seizures (occasionally)
  - Average age of death: 17 years

- Adult-onset (KUFS)
  - No ocular abnormalities
  - Benign; not fatal

FRIEDREICH'S ATAXIA

Friedreich's ataxia is an autosomal-recessive inherited disorder caused by a disturbance of pyruvate metabolism. Onset of symptoms is noted between 10 and 20 years of age.

- Ocular features
  - Pigmentary retinopathy
  - Vestibular nystagmus
  - Optic atrophy
  - Vertical gaze paresis

- Systemic features
  - Cerebellar ataxia
  - Absence of tendon reflexes
  - Scoliosis
  - Cardiomyopathy: Often the cause of death in the third to fourth decade of life

CARCINOMA-ASSOCIATED RETINOPATHY SYNDROME

Carcinoma-associated retinopathy (CAR) syndrome, also known as paraneoplastic retinopathy, is a visual paraneoplastic disorder in which autoantibodies against tumor antigen cross-react with retinal proteins, resulting in rod and cone photoreceptor dysfunction.

EPIDEMIOLOGY AND ETIOLOGY

- Age at presentation is variable.
- There is no gender preference.
- Associated malignancies include:
  - Small cell carcinoma of the lung (most common)
  - Gynecologic, breast, endocrine, or other visceral malignancies
- In CAR syndrome, autoantibodies cross-react with the protein recoverin, located within the photoreceptors.

HISTORY

- The typical presentation is severe, progressive, bilateral visual loss over a period of months, with relatively unremarkable fundus.
- Visual symptoms may precede diagnosis of the underlying malignancy.

CLINICAL SIGNS

- Cone dysfunction: As evidenced by:
  - Decreased visual acuity
  - Photosensitivity
  - Reduced color vision
  - Central scotoma
- Rod dysfunction: As evidenced by:

- Nyctalopia
- Prolonged dark adaptation
- Ring scotoma
- Fundus features
  - Early stages may be normal (**Fig. 5-26**)
  - Late finding: Narrow retinal arterioles
  - Retinal pigment epithelial mottling
  - Optic nerve pallor

ASSOCIATED CLINICAL FEATURES

- Systemic features of the underlying malignancy may or may not be present.

DIFFERENTIAL DIAGNOSIS

- Decreased vision from retinal cause and normal-appearing fundus
- Stargardt's disease
- Cone dystrophy
- Twig branch retinal vein occlusion
- Twig branch retinal artery occlusion
- Toxic retinopathy
- Reperfused central retinal artery occlusion
- Age, family and medication history, bilaterality, fluorescein angiography, and the electrophysiologic tests help to differentiate CAR syndrome from the preceding disorders.

DIAGNOSTIC EVALUATION

- Typical set of symptoms and signs
- Color vision: Reduced
- Visual fields: Typically, ring scotoma
- Dark adaptometry: Prolonged dark adaptation
- Electroretinography: Reduced amplitudes of both rod and cone responses

- Serum anti-recoverin antibodies
- Systemic oncologic evaluation

PROGNOSIS AND MANAGEMENT

- If photoreceptors are sufficiently damaged, visual functions are usually permanently altered.

- Various treatment measures have been tried, but their role in improving the visual prognosis remains to be proven. These measures include treatment of the underlying malignancy, steroids, plasmapheresis, and intravenous immunoglobulins.

FIGURE 5-26. **Carcinoma-associated retinopathy (CAR) syndrome. A.** Normal fundus but decreased vision. **B.** Severe and generalized visual field depression.

(*continued*)

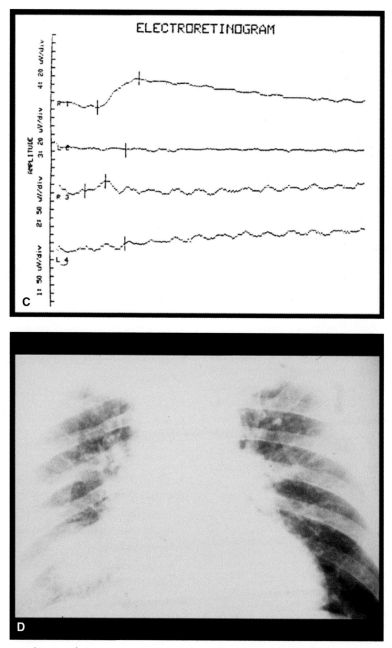

FIGURE 5-26. (*Continued*) **Carcinoma-associated retinopathy (CAR) syndrome. C.** Near completely extinguished electroretinogram. **D.** Mass lesion in the right lower lobe of the lung diagnosed as small cell carcinoma causing CAR syndrome. (Courtesy of Dr. William Tasman and the Retina Slide Collection, Wills Eye Hospital, Philadelphia, Pennsylvania, compiled by Dr. Tamara and Dr. Gordon Byrnes.)

Retinal and Choroidal Tumors

Franco M. Recchia

ASTROCYTIC HAMARTOMA

Astrocytic hamartoma is a congenital, minimally progressive, benign tumor arising from the glial cells of the retina and usually located around the optic disc. It is often associated with the systemic condition tuberous sclerosis (Bourneville's disease), occasionally with neurofibromatosis, but also occurs sporadically in otherwise normal individuals.

EPIDEMIOLOGY AND ETIOLOGY

- Most astrocytic hamartomas occur congenitally in association with tuberous sclerosis (TS), a familial phakomatosis characterized by the triad of seizures, mental retardation, and skin lesions. TS has an estimated incidence of 1 in 15,000 to 1 in 100,000 and exhibits autosomal-dominant inheritance. Roughly half of the patients with TS have astrocytic hamartomas. Causative genes have been identified on chromosomes 9q34 and 16p13.

HISTORY

- Patients with astrocytic hamartomas are usually asymptomatic. Visual field testing may reveal a scotoma in the area corresponding to the tumor.

IMPORTANT CLINICAL SIGNS

- The appearance of a retinal astrocytic hamartoma is principally of two types:
  - Smaller, noncalcified, flat, smooth tumor that appears as mild thickening of the nerve fiber layer
  - Larger, calcified, whitish-yellow nodular mass ("mulberry lesion")
- Aspects of both may be seen in the same lesion, as it is likely that calcification progresses slowly over many years (Fig. 6-1).
- Every patient with an astrocytic hamartoma of the retina or optic nerve *must* be evaluated for TS. Typical manifestations of TS include:

- Skin lesions (~95% incidence)

  ▶ Hypomelanotic macules: Oval ("ash-leaf"), polygonal, or punctate ("confetti") in shape. Usually present at birth and often the first presenting sign.

  ▶ Reddish-brown papular rash over the face (termed adenoma sebaceum, but actually angiofibromas), often mistaken for acne. Rarely present before a few years of age.

- Seizures (~90% incidence): Myoclonic spasms lasting 10 to 50 seconds; tend to become grand mal type later in life.

- Mental retardation (~60% incidence)

ASSOCIATED CLINICAL SIGNS

- Ocular: Occasionally, may produce vitreous hemorrhage, vitreous seeding, subretinal hemorrhage, or retinal detachment.

- Systemic (additional manifestations of TS): Ungual fibromas, pleural cysts (leading to spontaneous pneumothorax), renal angiomyolipoma, cardiac rhabdomyoma, and hamartomas of the liver, thyroid, pancreas, or testis may occur.

DIFFERENTIAL DIAGNOSIS

- Retinoblastoma (Rb)
- Myelinated nerve fibers

- Retinal granuloma
- Drusen of the optic disc
- Papillitis

DIAGNOSTIC EVALUATION

- Fluorescein angiography: The tumor appears relatively hypofluorescent in the arterial phase. Superficial fine blood vessels are seen during the venous phase. The tumor stains intensely and homogeneously in the late phases.

- B-scan Ultrasonography: A larger, calcified lesion often appears as a discrete, oval, solid mass with a sharp anterior border.

- Neuroimaging: Subependymal hamartomas, characteristic of TS, may be seen with computed tomography (CT) or magnetic resonance imaging (MRI).

PROGNOSIS AND MANAGEMENT

- The vast majority of retinal astrocytic hamartomas are asymptomatic and do not require treatment.

- Associated retinal detachment can often be treated with demarcating laser photocoagulation.

- Patients and family members should be examined regularly for manifestations of TS.

FIGURE 6-1. Astrocytic hamartoma. A peripapillary astrocytic hamartoma can be seen with classic mulberry calcification overlying an underlying smooth tumor. Patients and family members should be examined for tuberous sclerosis. Courtesy of Drs. Jerry and Carol Shields, Oncology Service, Wills Eye Hospital, Philadelphia, Pennsylvania.

RETINOBLASTOMA

R b is the most common intraocular malignancy of children. It may be familial but most often is sporadic in occurrence. The tumor arises from cells in the developing retina of one or both eyes as a result of mutations in the Rb) tumor-suppressor gene. Rb presents most often as a white intraocular mass with propensity for direct extension into the brain and almost certain mortality if untreated.

EPIDEMIOLOGY AND ETIOLOGY

- Rb occurs in approximately 1 in 15,000 live births. Most children are diagnosed at a mean of 18 months.

- No predilection for race or gender has been shown.

- Roughly two-thirds of the cases are unilateral, and one-third is bilateral. Unilateral cases are more likely to be diagnosed at an older age (mean of 24 months) and are most often nonfamilial (sporadic). Bilateral cases are diagnosed at a mean of 12 months, are usually familial, and are nearly always multifocal.

- Rb results from mutations or loss of both alleles of the Rb gene, located on chromosome 13q14. The Rb gene product appears to function as regulator of cellular proliferation through inhibitory effects on gene transcription at specific stages of the cell cycle. The timing of allelic inactivation determines whether the mutation is *germinal* (i.e., heritable by offspring of the affected child) or *somatic* (nonheritable). In germinal cases, a mutant allele is present before fertilization, most commonly as a result of inheritance from either parent. In somatic cases, both alleles are present and active at fertilization, and spontaneous mutations in each allele arise subsequently.

HISTORY

- A white pupillary reflex (leukokoria; Fig. 6-2) and strabismus are the two most common findings reported by parents. In fewer than 10% of cases is a family history known at the time of diagnosis.

IMPORTANT CLINICAL SIGNS

- Most patients present with leukokoria and strabismus. Small retinoblastomas appear as flat, translucent, white retinal lesions (Fig. 6-3A). With growth, the tumor appears more solid, elevated, and chalky-white, with overlying dilated tortuous blood vessels.

- Three growth patterns have been described.

  - Endophytic: The tumor grows from the retina inward to seed the vitreous cavity or anterior chamber.

  - Exophytic: The tumor grows from the retina outward to occupy the subretinal space, often causing an exudative retinal detachment (Fig. 6-3B).

  - Diffuse infiltrating: The least common form; this is characterized by shallow spread of tumor along the entire retina and into the vitreous and anterior chamber.

- Other important findings are iris neovascularization, which occurs in nearly one-fifth of all cases, and "pseudohypopyon" (settling of tumor and inflammatory cells in the anterior chamber).

ASSOCIATED CLINICAL SIGNS

- *Clear* lens
- Heterochromia iridis

- Spontaneous hyphema
- Extrascleral extension
- Pinealoblastoma ("trilateral retinoblastoma")

DIFFERENTIAL DIAGNOSIS

- Leukokoria
  - Coats' disease
  - Persistent fetal vasculature syndrome (formerly termed persistent hyperplastic primary vitreous, or PHPV)
  - Toxocariasis
  - Retinopathy of prematurity
  - Familial exudative vitreoretinopathy
  - Retinal astrocytoma
  - Cataract
  - Norrie's disease
  - Incontinentia pigmenti
- Vitreous seeding
  - Intraocular inflammation
  - Endophthalmitis
  - Vitreous hemorrhage
  - Leukemic infiltration

DIAGNOSTIC EVALUATION

- Detailed systemic evaluation and examination is required, as well as family history and ocular examination of parents, and complete examination of both eyes (often requiring anesthesia for complete visualization of the fundi with scleral depression).
- Ultrasonography: An elevated, rounded, intraocular mass is seen, with high internal reflectivity (calcification) and shadowing of sclera and soft tissue posterior to the lesion.
- CT is helpful in detecting intraocular calcification (present in roughly 80% of

retinoblastomas), assessing extraocular extension, and identifying the presence of pineal tumors.

- Fluorescein angiography reveals early arterial filling of the vessel feeding the tumor, leakage of dye from intrinsic tumor vessels, and late hyperfluorescence of the tumor.

PROGNOSIS

- Spontaneous regression is rare and leads to phthisis bulbi. Typically, if untreated, children die within 2 years of diagnosis. Early detection, coupled with improvements and promptness of treatment, has reduced the mortality rate to less than 10%. The main determinant for mortality is optic nerve invasion. For this reason, it is imperative to obtain as long a section of optic nerve as possible during enucleation.
- Prognostic factors for failure to preserve vision or to preserve the eye are larger tumor size, vitreous seeding, and macular involvement.
- Children with germinal Rb have an increased risk of developing other primary malignancies over the course of their lifetimes. These tumors include principally intracranial Rb, osteogenic sarcoma of the long bones, and sarcoma of soft tissues. The risk is estimated to be 20% within 25 years of treatment.

MANAGEMENT

- Children diagnosed with Rb should undergo evaluation for systemic involvement, including complete blood count, lumbar puncture, neuroimaging, and bone marrow biopsy. Genetic testing of the child and family members should be performed.
- Individual treatment varies according to number, size, and location of tumors, as

well as systemic status. Therapeutic options include cryotherapy, laser photocoagulation, enucleation, external-beam irradiation, plaque radiotherapy, chemotherapy, thermotherapy, and chemothermotherapy.

- Chemoreduction prior to definitive ocular treatment may be helpful in reducing the need for enucleation and reducing the rate of occurrence of pinealoblastoma.

- In familial cases, genetic counseling provides parents with important information regarding the probability of further occurrences. Patients with germinal Rb must be warned of the possibility of transmission to their offspring.

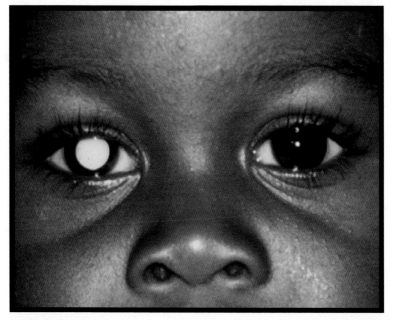

FIGURE 6-2. **Retinoblastoma.** This young boy has leukokoria and strabismus, the most common clinical presentation of retinoblastoma. Courtesy of Drs. Jerry and Carol Shields, Oncology Service, Wills Eye Hospital, Philadelphia, Pennsylvania.

FIGURE 6-3. Retinoblastoma. A. Focal retinoblastoma presenting as a macular intraretinal amelanotic tumor. **B.** Massive exophytic retinoblastoma with tumor behind the clear lens. Courtesy of Drs. Jerry and Carol Shields, Oncology Service, Wills Eye Hospital, Philadelphia, Pennsylvania.

RETINAL CAPILLARY HEMANGIOMA

Originally termed *angiomatosis retinae,* retinal capillary hemangioma is a benign vascular tumor of variable size located in the retina or adjacent to the optic disc. Usually diagnosed by the fourth decade, it may be the first manifestation of von Hippel–Lindau (VHL) disease, a familial cancer syndrome with which it is commonly associated.

EPIDEMIOLOGY AND ETIOLOGY

- This tumor may occur in a sporadic or hereditary fashion. Retinal capillary hemangioma occurs in up to 80% of patients with VHL syndrome and is often the first manifestation, diagnosed at a mean age of 25 years.
- The VHL syndrome has an estimated prevalence of 1 in 40,000 and is possibly more common in whites. It exhibits dominant inheritance and has variable phenotypes within families.
- Mean survival of patients with VHL is 41 years of age.
- VHL syndrome is caused by mutations in the VHL gene, a tumor-suppressor gene located on chromosome 3p25. The VHL gene product regulates the expression and function of hypoxia-responsive angiogenic factors [e.g., vascular endothelial growth factor (VEGF)].

HISTORY

- Capillary hemangiomas may be diagnosed incidentally or in patients suspected of having VHL syndrome. The tumors may be asymptomatic or may produce painless visual impairment from vitreous hemorrhage, macular pucker, or retinal detachment.

IMPORTANT CLINICAL SIGNS

- Retinal capillary hemangioma: Usually located peripherally and well circumscribed. Initially appears as a yellow-red dot with a minimally dilated "feeding" arteriole or draining venule (**Fig. 6-4**). With growth, appears orange-red with more prominently dilated afferent and efferent vessels. May have associated exudation, subretinal fluid, or preretinal fibrosis.
- Juxtapapillary capillary hemangioma: Orange-red in color, but less well circumscribed. It often lacks feeder vessels.
- VHL syndrome: Hemangio-blastomas of the cerebellum and spinal cord, renal cell carcinoma, or pheochromocytoma.

ASSOCIATED CLINICAL SIGNS

- Retinal detachment and, rarely, neovascular glaucoma may complicate capillary hemangioma.
- Hemangiomas of the adrenal glands, lungs, and liver, and multiple cysts of the pancreas and kidneys have been observed in some patients with VHL syndrome.

DIFFERENTIAL DIAGNOSIS

- Retinal capillary hemangioma
  - Other tumors: Retinal cavernous hemangioma, racemose hemangioma, choroidal melanoma, and astrocytic hamartoma
  - Vascular diseases: Coats' disease, retinal arterial macroaneurysm, familial exudative vitreoretinopathy, and exudative macular degeneration
  - *N.B.*: A distinction has been made between the retinal angioma of VHL

syndrome and an acquired, nonhereditary entity occurring in older patients and termed *vasoproliferative retinal tumor*. This latter condition is usually located in the inferotemporal peripheral fundus and lacks markedly dilated feeder vessels.

- Optic disc hemangioma
  - Papillitis
  - Optic disc granuloma
  - Optic disc glioma

DIAGNOSTIC EVALUATION

- Ocular: Fluorescein angiography is the most helpful ancillary study. In the arterial phase, a prominent, dilated feeder arteriole may be seen. The tumor appears hyperfluorescent early and remains so through the late phases, sometimes leaking dye into the vitreous. Ultrasonography may be helpful in diagnosing lesions of greater than 1 mm and demonstrates acoustic solidity throughout the lesion.

- Systemic: All patients with retinal capillary hemangioma, as well as relatives, should be evaluated for VHL syndrome. Genetic testing for mutations in the VHL gene is available.

PROGNOSIS AND MANAGEMENT

- The natural history is variable, with both progressive enlargement and spontaneous regression having been reported. Visual prognosis is highly variable and depends on tumor location, size, and associated complications, especially those that involve the macula.

- In patients with VHL syndrome, risk of developing associated tumors increases with age. Morbidity and mortality are related to these associated tumors. Median survival is less than 50 years, with renal carcinoma as the leading cause of death.

- Treatment is recommended for tumors with documented growth or effects on visual function. The goal of treatment is to induce resolution of exudation or subretinal fluid. Laser photocoagulation is reserved for smaller tumors (less than 2 mm in diameter). Larger tumors are best treated with cryotherapy or plaque radiotherapy. Vitreoretinal surgery, and, rarely, enucleation may be necessary for patients with advanced or uncontrollable pathology.

- Patients with VHL syndrome and their relatives should be examined regularly for life. This includes regular testing for urine catecholamines, CT and ultrasonography of the kidneys, and MRI of the brain.

FIGURE 6-4. **Retinal capillary hemangioma.** Note the dilated feeding retinal arteriole (*arrow*) and the segmented draining retinal vein (*arrowhead*) with associated macular edema, premacular fibrosis, and lipid exudation. These lesions may be the first manifestation of von Hippel–Lindau disease. Courtesy of Drs. Jerry and Carol Shields, Oncology Service, Wills Eye Hospital, Philadelphia, Pennsylvania.

RETINAL CAVERNOUS HEMANGIOMA

Retinal cavernous hemangioma is a benign, rarely progressive, vascular tumor of the retina or optic disc characterized by a collection of venous aneurysms. It may be associated with similar vascular anomalies of the skin and central nervous system (CNS).

EPIDEMIOLOGY AND ETIOLOGY

- Tumor occurrence is mostly sporadic.
- Small pedigrees of patients with cavernous hemangioma as part of a dominantly inherited oculoneurocutaneous syndrome have been reported.

HISTORY

- Patients are usually asymptomatic, but the tumor may produce painless visual loss.
- A hereditary component may be noted.

IMPORTANT CLINICAL SIGNS

- A cluster of dark-red, intraretinal aneurysms is located along a retinal venule, appearing as a "cluster of grapes" arising from the inner retinal surface (Fig. 6-5). Often there is overlying gray fibroglial tissue. Usually the tumor does *not* have associated exudation or a feeding arteriole.

ASSOCIATED CLINICAL SIGNS

- Vitreous hemorrhage occurs in up to 10% of cases.

- There may also be cutaneous vascular malformations.
- Cavernous hemangiomas of the midbrain or cerebellum may produce seizures or subarachnoid hemorrhage.

DIFFERENTIAL DIAGNOSIS

- Capillary hemangioma
- Acquired vasoproliferative tumor
- Racemose hemangioma
- Coats' disease

DIAGNOSTIC EVALUATION

- Fluorescein angiography produces a typical pattern: The lesion is hypofluorescent in the early arterial phase and exhibits slow hyperfluorescence during the late venous phase as dye enters the venous channels. A fluorescein–blood interface may be seen within the aneurysms in the late phases of the angiogram.

PROGNOSIS AND MANAGEMENT

- Most cavernous hemangiomas do not enlarge and can be managed with periodic observation.
- The main complication is vitreous hemorrhage, although this rarely causes permanent visual loss.
- Tumors causing recurrent vitreous hemorrhage may be treated with cryotherapy, laser photocoagulation, or plaque radiotherapy.

FIGURE 6-5. **Retinal cavernous hemangioma.** Note the "cluster of grapes" appearance of these intraretinal aneurysms (inset). There is a lack of exudation, and surface gray retinal fibrous tissue is noted. Courtesy of Drs. Jerry and Carol Shields, Oncology Service, Wills Eye Hospital, Philadelphia, Pennsylvania.

CONGENITAL HYPERTROPHY OF THE RETINAL PIGMENT EPITHELIUM

DEFINITION

Congenital hypertrophy of the retinal pigment epithelium (CHRPE) is a benign, asymptomatic condition, consisting of one or more well-demarcated, pigmented, flat, nonprogressive lesions, usually found in the equatorial or peripheral fundus. In rare instances, multifocal lesions may be associated with familial colonic polyposis.

EPIDEMIOLOGY AND ETIOLOGY

- The condition is probably congenital.
- It occurs with equal frequency in blacks and whites.

HISTORY

- Patients are usually asymptomatic. Often the disorder is noted as an incidental finding during ophthalmoscopy.

IMPORTANT CLINICAL SIGNS

- Two forms have been described.
  - Solitary: Unilateral, deeply pigmented, flat, circular lesion measuring 1 to 6 mm in diameter. Usually sharply demarcated, the lesion may be solid black, or ringed with a small border of hypopigmentation. Lacunar areas of depigmentation within the lesion may be seen (Fig. 6-6).
  - Multifocal: Also termed congenital grouped pigmentation or "bear tracks." Groups of 3 to 30 small (0.1 to 2 mm) lesions typically appear in one sector of the midperipheral retina. Usually they lack the internal lacunae and hypopigmented halo of the solitary form.

- Multifocal fundus lesions resembling CHRPE have been reported in close association with Gardner's syndrome (Fig. 6-7), a familial condition of colonic polyps and extraintestinal osteomas and fibromas with invariable progression to colonic cancer. The lesions associated with Gardner's syndrome, however, are bilateral, have irregular borders, and are often scattered in the fundus.

DIFFERENTIAL DIAGNOSIS

- Malignant choroidal melanoma
- Choroidal nevus
- Combined hamartoma of the retina and retinal pigment epithelium (RPE)

DIAGNOSTIC EVALUATION

- Diagnosis is based on typical ophthalmoscopic features. By fluorescein angiography, the tumor exhibits persistent hypofluorescence. Lacunar areas are seen as hyperfluorescent, consistent with depigmentation of the RPE.

PROGNOSIS AND MANAGEMENT

- Most CHRPE lesions are nonprogressive and require only periodic examination. In rare instances, mild enlargement may occur.
- Patients with bilateral lesions suggestive of those seen in Gardner's syndrome should be referred for colonoscopy.

FIGURE 6-6. Congenital hypertrophy of the retinal pigment epithelium. Note the sharp, discrete borders of the lesion as well as the lacunar areas of depigmentation (*arrow*) within the lesion. Courtesy of Drs. Jerry and Carol Shields, Oncology Service, Wills Eye Hospital, Philadelphia, Pennsylvania.

FIGURE 6-7. **Pigmented fundus lesion, Gardner's syndrome.** Pigmented lesion associated with Gardner's syndrome and familial gastrointestinal cancer. A depigmented "tail" (*arrowheads*) is noted adjacent to the pigmented fundus lesion (insets). Courtesy of Drs. Jerry and Carol Shields, Oncology Service, Wills Eye Hospital, Philadelphia, Pennsylvania.

COMBINED HAMARTOMA OF THE RETINA AND RETINAL PIGMENT EPITHELIUM

Combined hamartoma of the retina and RPE is a benign, slightly elevated, partially pigmented tumor located around the optic nerve or in the peripheral fundus. It is composed histologically of proliferated glial cells, fibrovascular tissue, and pigment epithelial cells.

EPIDEMIOLOGY AND ETIOLOGY

- The tumor is often diagnosed by early adulthood. The preponderance of cases in infants and young children suggests that the lesion may be congenital.

- An association of combined hamartomas, usually macular and sometimes bilateral, has been seen with neurofibromatosis (most commonly type 2).

HISTORY

- In cases of juxtafoveal lesions, there is painless visual loss from epimacular membrane traction or subretinal exudation.

IMPORTANT CLINICAL SIGNS

- Juxtapapillary variant: Ill-defined, elevated, charcoal-gray mass adjacent to, or overlying, the optic disc. A gray-white membrane overlying the tumor causes stretching of retinal blood vessels and retinal striae, often involving the macula (Fig. 6-8).

- Peripheral variant: Slightly elevated, pigmented ridge concentric to the optic disc. There is dragging of dilated retinal vessels toward the lesion by the overlying membrane.

ASSOCIATED CLINICAL SIGNS

- Choroidal neovascularization
- Vitreous hemorrhage
- Manifestations of neurofibromatosis type 2 (bilateral acoustic neuromas, brain meningiomas, spinal cord schwannomas, posterior subcapsular cataracts)

DIFFERENTIAL DIAGNOSIS

- Choroidal melanoma
- Choroidal nevus
- Reactive hyperplasia of the RPE
- Melanocytoma
- When lightly pigmented and occurring in children, may be mistaken for Rb or toxocariasis

DIAGNOSTIC EVALUATION

- Diagnosis is based on ophthalmoscopic features. Fluorescein angiography reveals multiple, dilated, fine blood vessels within the tumor, which may become hyperfluorescent as the angiogram progresses.

PROGNOSIS AND MANAGEMENT

- Since lesions are usually not progressive, regular observation is appropriate. However, contraction of overlying fibroglial tissue leads to macular distortion, secondary retinoschisis, and retinal holes.

- In cases of visual loss, vitrectomy and membrane stripping may be performed, but visual recovery is limited.

FIGURE 6-8. **Combined hamartoma of the retina and retinal pigment epithelium.** This is an example of the juxtapapillary variant of the lesion. The edge of an apparent membrane is noted most prominently on the nasal aspect of the lesion. There is marked distortion and tortuosity of the involved retinal vasculature. Courtesy of Drs. Jerry and Carol Shields, Oncology Service, Wills Eye Hospital, Philadelphia, Pennsylvania.

CHOROIDAL NEVUS

Choroidal nevus is a common, benign tumor of the posterior fundus. Although usually flat or minimally elevated, and gray or brown in appearance, it may show variable degrees of pigmentation.

EPIDEMIOLOGY

- Prevalence in the general population is estimated to be 1% to 6%. The tumor occurs much more commonly in whites.

HISTORY

- Patients are usually asymptomatic, and the tumor is generally discovered incidentally during routine ophthalmoscopy.

- Vision may be reduced from extension of associated subretinal fluid into the macula, or from an associated serous retinal detachment.

IMPORTANT CLINICAL SIGNS

- The tumor is most often slate gray or brown in color, but it may be heterogeneously pigmented or even amelanotic (pale yellow).

- Choroidal nevi are usually 1 to 5 mm in diameter, flat or minimally elevated (less than 2 mm in anteroposterior dimension), with ill-defined margins.

- Drusen overlying the tumor are common and signify chronicity of the lesion (Fig. 6-9).

- Alterations of the overlying RPE include pigment clumping and fibrous metaplasia (yellow-white plaques). "Orange pigment" at the level of the RPE represents aggregates of macrophages containing lipofuscin granules and may suggest growth or malignant transformation of the nevus.

ASSOCIATED CLINICAL SIGNS

- Serous detachment of the neurosensory retina or RPE
- Choroidal neovascularization

DIFFERENTIAL DIAGNOSIS

- Pigmented lesion
  - Choroidal melanoma
  - Congenital hypertrophy of the RPE
  - Combined hamartoma of the retina and RPE
  - Subretinal hemorrhage
- Amelanotic lesion
  - Circumscribed choroidal hemangioma
  - Choroidal osteoma
  - Choroidal metastasis
  - Inflammatory lesion

DIAGNOSTIC EVALUATION

- Diagnosis is based on characteristic ophthalmoscopic features. Fluorescein angiography, although not specific for choroidal nevus, may provide confirmatory evidence. Areas of deep pigmentation are hypofluorescent, whereas areas of overlying RPE alteration will appear hyperfluorescent.

- Ultrasonography may be helpful for establishing baseline thickness.

PROGNOSIS AND MANAGEMENT

- All small choroidal melanocytic tumors have the potential for malignant transformation and metastasis. Risk factors for growth include greater thickness (larger than 2 mm), proximity to the optic disc, orange pigment on the surface of the tumor, and presence of subretinal fluid. The chance of growth of small, flat ("nonsuspicious") lesions lacking these clinical features is less than 5%.

- Management consists of baseline photographs and regular examination to establish quiescence or growth of the nevus. Serial photographs, ultrasonography, and more frequent examinations are indicated in cases of suspected growth.

FIGURE 6-9. **Choroidal nevus.** This is a minimally elevated choroidal pigmented lesion with overlying drusen (*arrow*). No orange pigment or submacular fluid suggestive of potential transformation of a malignant choroidal melanoma is noted. Courtesy of Drs. Jerry and Carol Shields, Oncology Service, Wills Eye Hospital, Philadelphia, Pennsylvania.

CHOROIDAL MELANOMA

Choroidal melanoma is the most common primary intraocular malignancy, occurring most often in white adults. Dome- or mushroom-shaped, this variably pigmented mass arises from the choroid of one eye. It has a propensity for metastasis to the liver.

EPIDEMIOLOGY AND ETIOLOGY

- The incidence is 1 in 2000 to 1 in 2500 in Caucasians. In the United States, choroidal melanoma is nearly ten times more common in whites than in African Americans.
- There is no gender predilection.
- The tumor is uncommon in people younger than 30, but incidence increases with age and the average age at diagnosis is in the sixth decade.
- Risk factors may include prolonged exposure to ultraviolet light, congenital oculodermal melanocytosis (nevus of Ota), and family history.
- The tumor arises from dendritic melanocytes of the choroid. Histopathologically, there are two major categories of cells: spindle cells and epithelioid cells.
- Rare associated karyotypic abnormalities have been reported, most commonly alterations of chromosome 3.

HISTORY

- The malignancy is usually asymptomatic and painless.
- Visual effects include blurred vision, floaters, photopsia, and visual field defects.

IMPORTANT CLINICAL SIGNS

- The tumor appears as a dome-shaped, elevated choroidal mass, typically confined to the subretinal space. About 20% of choroidal melanomas break through Bruch's membrane and take on a characteristic mushroom shape.
- Color varies from brown to gray to pale yellow (amelanotic), with overlying clumps of orange pigment, representing collections of lipofuscin (**Fig. 6-10**).
- Associated subretinal fluid, usually surrounding the base of the lesion, may be noted, and the tumor may lead to total serous retinal detachment.

ASSOCIATED CLINICAL SIGNS

- Vitreous hemorrhage
- Subretinal hemorrhage
- Choroidal neovascularization
- Extrascleral extension with orbital invasion

DIFFERENTIAL DIAGNOSIS

- Choroidal nevus
- Choroidal metastasis
- Combined hamartoma of the retina and RPE
- Congenital hypertrophy of the RPE (CHRPE)
- Circumscribed choroidal hemangioma, reactive hyperplasia of the RPE
- Bilateral diffuse uveal melanocytic proliferation
- Choroidal osteoma

DIAGNOSTIC EVALUATION

• Diagnosis is based on ophthalmoscopic features. Ultrasonography reveals an acoustically hollow, dome-shaped or mushroom-shaped mass with low internal reflectivity. Ultrasonographic measurements of tumor thickness are valuable in determination of doses for radiotherapy, as well as for serial evaluation following treatment.

• Fluorescein angiography of small choroidal tumors shows early mottled hyperfluorescence of the tumor with progressive staining in the late phases. Large tumors display filling of large intrinsic vessels in the venous phase, with diffuse late staining.

PROGNOSIS

• Overall, 5-year survival for patients with choroidal melanoma is about 80%. Median survival is about 7 years. Prognosis for survival depends on a variety of factors, including age at diagnosis, intraocular location, extent of metastasis, tumor size, and tumor cell type. The 5-year mortality for patients with epithelioid melanomas is 42%; for those with spindle cell tumors, 10%. The 5-year mortality for patients with tumors with largest basal tumor diameter (LTD) greater than 15 mm is nearly 50%; for those with LTD less than 10 mm, under 20%.

• Risk factors for metastasis include documented growth, proximity to the optic disc, and greater tumor thickness. Nearly one-half of the patients with metastatic choroidal melanoma die within 1 year of treatment. There appears to be no difference in mortality in patients treated initially with enucleation when compared with those treated with iodine-125 plaque radiotherapy.

• Higher risk for metastasis and mortality appears to be associated with specific patterns of gene expression, which can be determined through analysis of tumor tissue.

MANAGEMENT

Ocular

• The primary goal of treatment of choroidal melanoma is prevention of metastasis. Choice of specific modality depends on tumor size, location, and the patient's systemic and psychological status.

• Enucleation remains the standard treatment for large melanomas (greater than 12 mm in LTD and 8 mm in thickness). Other options for smaller tumors include transpupillary thermotherapy (TTT), radiotherapy (plaque brachytherapy or proton-beam irradiation), and local resection (reserved for anterior lesions). Observation is appropriate for small tumors with little evidence of growth.

• Patients should be evaluated regularly with careful funduscopy, serial fundus photographs, and ultrasonography.

Systemic

• The vast majority (~98%) of patients have no discernible metastasis at the time of diagnosis of their choroidal melanoma.

• Baseline systemic evaluation should be performed in every patient, under the direction of a medical oncologist. Assessment typically includes complete blood count, liver enzyme panel, chest roentgenogram, and imaging (i.e., CT or ultrasound) of the abdomen.

• Measurement of liver enzymes should be performed regularly along with ophthalmoscopy.

FIGURE 6-10. Choroidal melanoma. A. A large, elevated, pigmented choroidal mass surrounding the temporal aspect of the optic disc is appreciated with overlying orange pigment. The primary goal of treatment of choroidal melanoma is prevention of systemic metastases. **B.** A large, elevated, pigmented choroidal mass with subretinal fluid and orange pigment. Orange pigment may represent macrophage ingestion of lipofuscin pigment and reflect tumor activity. Courtesy of Drs. Jerry and Carol Shields, Oncology Service, Wills Eye Hospital, Philadelphia, Pennsylvania.

CHOROIDAL MELANOCYTOMA

Choroidal melanocytoma is a benign, minimally progressive, deeply pigmented tumor occurring at or around the optic nerve. It is probably a variant of choroidal nevus.

EPIDEMIOLOGY

• Blacks and whites are affected equally. Malignant melanomas, by contrast, occur much less frequently in black patients.

HISTORY

• Patients are usually asymptomatic.

• Visual loss may occur in rare instances of tumor growth or retinal vascular obstruction.

• No inheritance pattern has been recognized.

IMPORTANT CLINICAL SIGNS

• Characteristically, this charcoal gray or gray-black tumor is located on or adjacent to the optic disc, with both a deep choroidal component and superficial extension into the nerve fiber layer (**Fig. 6-11**).

• It is usually unilateral.

• A relative afferent papillary defect (RAPD) may be seen in up to 30% of cases.

ASSOCIATED CLINICAL SIGNS

• The uninvolved area of the optic disc may become acutely edematous with an associated decline in vision.

• Rarely, neovascular glaucoma secondary to vascular obstruction may occur.

DIFFERENTIAL DIAGNOSIS

• Juxtapapillary choroidal melanoma
• Choroidal nevus
• Hyperplasia of the RPE
• Combined hamartoma of the retina and RPE

DIAGNOSTIC EVALUATION

• Diagnosis is based on characteristic ophthalmoscopic features.

• Regular examinations and serial fundus photographs are essential for documentation of growth or malignant transformation.

PROGNOSIS AND MANAGEMENT

• The patient is followed by observation.

• Roughly 15% of melanocytomas exhibit small degrees of enlargement. However, malignant transformation is possible and is often heralded by more rapid growth and visual changes. In such cases, enucleation of the affected eye should be considered.

FIGURE 6-11. **Choroidal melanocytoma.** Note the dark brown lesion involving the optic disc. There are feathery edges to the lesion. A small percentage (~15%) of melanocytomas will demonstrate some growth; malignant transformation is rare but has been reported. Courtesy of Drs. Jerry and Carol Shields, Oncology Service, Wills Eye Hospital, Philadelphia, Pennsylvania.

CHOROIDAL METASTASIS

Choroidal metastasis is the most common intraocular malignancy, visible ophthalmoscopically in up to 1% of patients with systemic malignancy (most commonly arising from the lungs or breasts). Clinically it is apparent as an amelanotic, shallow, round or oval choroidal mass posterior to the equator. Choroidal metastasis is usually unilateral but may be multifocal and bilateral. It is the presenting sign of metastatic malignancy in up to one-third of the patients.

EPIDEMIOLOGY AND ETIOLOGY

- There is a cumulative lifetime incidence of 1 in 400 to 1 in 1000 Americans.

- At autopsy, microscopic intraocular lesions are detectable in 5% to 10% of patients with systemic malignancy; of these, 10% have clinically apparent lesions. The increasing incidence is likely attributable to increased survival of patients with cancer, improved detection, and greater awareness.

- The most common primary malignancy is breast carcinoma in women and lung carcinoma in men. In patients with no known primary site at the time of diagnosis, systemic evaluation leads to diagnosis of lung carcinoma in one-third of the patients and breast carcinoma in one-tenth of the patients. Known primary sites other than breasts and lungs comprise less than 10% of cases with choroidal metastasis. In one-half of the patients, however, a primary site is not discovered.

- Tumors are overwhelmingly carcinomas, rarely sarcomas. Spread is hematogenous. Cytologic findings are consistent with the tumor of origin.

HISTORY

- Blurred vision (usually painless) is reported in 80% of patients. Floaters and visual field defects are other symptoms, along with eye pain (5% to 15%). A history of malignancy is noted in 65% to 75% of patients.

IMPORTANT CLINICAL SIGNS

- The tumor appears as a round or oval, placoid, minimally elevated choroidal mass that is variable in color. It is unifocal and unilateral in roughly two-thirds of the cases. Metastases from breast and lung are typically pale yellow, whereas those from cutaneous melanoma are dark gray or brown (Fig. 6-12). Other tumors with characteristic coloration include metastatic renal cell and thyroid carcinoma (typically orange-red) and metastatic carcinoid tumors (typically pink or yellow-orange).

- Typically the tumor is located posterior to the equator (greater than 90%); it is predominantly macular in roughly 10%.

- Tumor growth may result in disc edema and serous retinal detachment.

ASSOCIATED CLINICAL SIGNS

- Conjunctival injection
- Hyperopic shift
- Neovascular glaucoma

DIFFERENTIAL DIAGNOSIS

- Amelanotic choroidal melanoma
- Circumscribed choroidal hemangioma

- Retinal astrocytoma
- Choroidal osteoma
- Intraocular lymphoma
- Sclerochoroidal calcification
- Central serous chorioretinopathy
- Choroidal granuloma
- Posterior scleritis
- Vitelliform dystrophy

DIAGNOSTIC EVALUATION

- Fluorescein angiography of carcinoma metastatic to the choroid shows early hypo-fluorescence of the lesion with a relative paucity of intrinsic vessels, and diffuse hyper-fluorescence of the tumor in the late phases of the study. Indocyanine green angiography may demonstrate additional, smaller choroidal tumors.

- Ultrasonography is most helpful for elevated tumors; they appear hyperechoic (bright) with high internal reflectivity. Fine-needle aspiration biopsy may be helpful, especially in patients with no known malignancy.

PROGNOSIS

- Most metastatic tumors are relentlessly progressive and tend to grow faster than primary choroidal malignancies. If untreated, bullous retinal detachment can lead to

blindness and secondary angle-closure glaucoma.

- Optic disc edema causes profound and often irreversible visual loss. Factors related to the preservation of vision and eye structures include number and size of tumors, proximity to the optic nerve and fovea, and responsiveness to therapy.

- Survival is related to effective treatment and remission of systemic disease. Patients with choroidal metastasis from breast carcinoma tend to survive longer than patients with choroidal metastases from other sites.

MANAGEMENT

- Ocular: Choroidal metastases are most often treated with external-beam radiotherapy, chemotherapy, hormonal therapy, or a combination. Single, smaller tumors may be treated effectively with plaque radiotherapy.

- Systemic: Patients with systemic disease should be referred to a medical oncologist. Management of patients with a known primary extraocular malignancy requires a staging evaluation appropriate for the primary tumor. Patients with no known primary site at time of diagnosis are evaluated with a thorough physical examination (with attention to breasts and lymph nodes), mammography, chest roentgenogram, CT of the chest, abdomen, and pelvis, and bone and PET scans.

FIGURE 6-12. Choroidal metastasis. A. Metastatic lung cancer presents as an amelanotic choroidal lesion (*arrow*) superior to the optic disc. Most choroidal metastases occur posterior to the equator. They may be unifocal or multifocal. (Courtesy of Drs. Jerry and Carol Shields, Oncology Service, Wills Eye Hospital, Philadelphia, Pennsylvania.) **B. Choroidal metastasis to iris.** Metastatic breast cancer presents initially to the patient as an amelanotic iris mass.

CHOROIDAL HEMANGIOMA

Choroidal hemangioma is a benign vascular tumor that occurs in two forms: circumscribed (discrete) and diffuse. The circumscribed variant is a well-defined, orange-red, dome-shaped mass, usually occurring in the posterior fundus and diagnosed by the fourth decade of life. The diffuse variant is characteristically associated with Sturge–Weber syndrome (encephalotrigeminal angiomatosis) and is diagnosed at a younger age. It gives a markedly asymmetric, bright red reflex to the fundus of the involved eye.

EPIDEMIOLOGY

- Circumscribed type: Sporadic, usually diagnosed in third or fourth decade. May be worsened by pregnancy. Usually unilateral.
- Diffuse type: Diagnosed in childhood. Occurs in roughly one-third of the patients with Sturge–Weber syndrome. Usually unilateral and ipsilateral to the characteristic facial hemangioma (nevus flammeus, or "port-wine stain"), but may be bilateral and associated with bilateral facial hemangiomas.

HISTORY

- Patients may be asymptomatic.
- Visual impairment is usually painless and results from hyperopic shift (in cases of submacular tumor) or subretinal fluid.

IMPORTANT CLINICAL SIGNS

- Circumscribed type
  - Discrete, slightly elevated, orange-red mass arising in the posterior choroid

- Serous retinal detachment in two-thirds of the cases
  - Overlying RPE metaplasia or retinoschisis (Fig. 6-13)
- Diffuse type
  - Bright red color involving a large section (more than 50%) of the fundus
  - Tortuosity of overlying retinal vessels
  - Shifting subretinal fluid
- Manifestations of Sturge–Weber syndrome include facial nevus flammeus (100% of patients), cerebral abnormalities, and intracranial calcifications. Asymmetric cupping of the optic nerve (due to congenital glaucoma) occurs, particularly in cases of nevus flammeus involving the ipsilateral upper eyelid.

ASSOCIATED CLINICAL SIGNS

- Choroidal neovascularization (circumscribed type)
- Retinitis pigmentosa-like changes (diffuse type)

DIFFERENTIAL DIAGNOSIS

- Central serous retinopathy
- Amelanotic choroidal melanoma
- Choroidal metastasis
- Choroidal inflammation

DIAGNOSTIC EVALUATION

- Fluorescein angiography and indocyanine green angiography reveal early hyperfluorescence corresponding to filling of choroidal vessels feeding the tumor.
- B-scan ultrasonography demonstrates a dome-shaped elevation in the case of a circumscribed hemangioma and marked choroidal thickening in cases of diffuse tumors.

PROGNOSIS AND MANAGEMENT

- Management consists of observation as long as the patients are asymptomatic. In cases of macular involvement or extensive retinal detachment, visual impairment is inevitable, and treatment is indicated.

- Treatment consists of radiation therapy (external-beam, cobalt-60 brachytherapy, or proton-beam irradiation). Delimiting laser photocoagulation, external drainage, or scleral buckling is indicated for retinal detachment.

FIGURE 6-13. **Choroidal hemangioma, circumscribed type.** A macular choroidal hemangioma demonstrates submacular fluid and overlying retinal pigment epithelial metaplasia (*arrow*). This lesion is often confused with central serous retinopathy. Courtesy of Drs. Jerry and Carol Shields, Oncology Service, Wills Eye Hospital, Philadelphia, Pennsylvania.

INTRAOCULAR LYMPHOMA

Intraocular lymphoma is a malignant, indolent, often bilateral, lymphocytic proliferation with diffuse infiltration of the posterior segment that occurs in two forms: (1) arising primarily from the eye or CNS; or (2) systemic, usually visceral, lymphoma, metastatic to the uvea. Most often it affects older patients and is associated with CNS lymphoma. Intraocular lymphoma was formerly termed *reticulum cell sarcoma*.

EPIDEMIOLOGY AND ETIOLOGY

• Usually intraocular lymphoma affects immunocompetent patients in their sixth to seventh decade. It is bilateral in up to 90% of cases. A more aggressive form is seen in patients who are severely immunocompromised, most commonly from the acquired immunodeficiency syndrome (AIDS).

• Intraocular lymphoma is the presenting sign of CNS lymphoma in 80% of patients, but may precede CNS involvement by up to 10 years (mean of 2 years). The incidence appears to be increasing, possibly as a result of more widespread immunosuppression or improved diagnosis.

• Most often the lymphoma is a large-cell B lymphocytic (i.e., non-Hodgkin) tumor. It is thought to arise from cells of the retina, RPE, brain, meninges, and spinal cord.

HISTORY

• Patients have a history of floaters and painless visual loss.

• Chronic, unremitting vitritis that is unresponsive to corticosteroids occurs, along with neurologic impairment.

IMPORTANT CLINICAL SIGNS

• Vitreous inflammation
• Multiple, yellow-white lesions deep to the retina that progressively enlarge and coalesce
• Overlying pigmentary alterations

ASSOCIATED CLINICAL SIGNS

• Anterior uveitis
• Retinal vasculitis, leading to vascular obstruction (Fig. 6-14)
• Optic disc edema

DIFFERENTIAL DIAGNOSIS

• Vitritis
  ▪ Amyloidosis
  ▪ Old vitreous hemorrhage
  ▪ Senile vitritis
• Retinal infiltrates and vasculitis
  ▪ Toxoplasmosis
  ▪ Cytomegalovirus retinitis
  ▪ Acute retinal necrosis
  ▪ Sarcoidosis
• Subretinal infiltrates
  ▪ Multifocal choroiditis
  ▪ Acute posterior multifocal placoid pigment epitheliopathy
  ▪ Multiple evanescent white dot syndrome
  ▪ Fundus flavimaculatus
  ▪ Choroidal granuloma
  ▪ Amelanotic choroidal melanoma
  ▪ Choroidal metastasis
  ▪ Bilateral diffuse uveal melanocytic proliferation

DIAGNOSTIC EVALUATION

• In the absence of known CNS disease, vitreous biopsy (through either fine-needle aspiration or pars plana vitrectomy) has the greatest diagnostic yield. Multiple vitreous specimens may be needed.

PROGNOSIS AND MANAGEMENT

• All patients with intraocular lymphoma should be evaluated for CNS and systemic involvement, by neurologic examination, neuroimaging (thin-section magnetic resonance imaging), lumbar puncture, and bone marrow biopsy.

• Untreated, most patients die within a few years of diagnosis. Patients with disease limited to the eye may be treated with external-beam irradiation only. Adjunct chemotherapy and corticosteroids prolong survival to a median of 41 months (with 22% disease-free at 5 years), but do not decrease the risk of subsequent CNS involvement.

• Ocular relapse, especially within the first year after treatment, is common.

FIGURE 6-14. **Intraocular lymphoma.** Hazy photograph demonstrating vitritis and intraretinal invasion of lymphoma with associated hemorrhagic retinal vasculitis. Courtesy of Drs. Jerry and Carol Shields, Oncology Service, Wills Eye Hospital, Philadelphia, Pennsylvania.

CHOROIDAL OSTEOMA

Choroidal osteoma is a rare, benign choroidal tumor composed of mature bone, occurring most commonly in the posterior pole of one eye of healthy young women.

EPIDEMIOLOGY AND ETIOLOGY

- The tumor most often affects women younger than 30 years of age.
- It is unilateral in 75% of cases and usually sporadic, but rare familial cases have been reported.

HISTORY

- Patients are usually asymptomatic.
- Diminished visual acuity or metamorphopsia are caused by macular involvement by the tumor or by associated choroidal neovascularization.

IMPORTANT CLINICAL SIGNS

- The tumor is most often adjacent to, or surrounding, the optic disc. It appears pale yellow to orange in color and is minimally elevated (usually less than 2 mm in thickness). Overlying clumping of brown, gray, or orange pigment may be noted (Fig. 6-15).

ASSOCIATED CLINICAL SIGNS

- Choroidal neovascularization
- Serous retinal detachment

DIFFERENTIAL DIAGNOSIS

- Amelanotic choroidal melanoma
- Carcinoma metastatic to the choroid
- Circumscribed choroidal hemangioma
- Disciform scar of age-related macular degeneration
- Idiopathic sclerochoroidal calcification

DIAGNOSTIC EVALUATION

- Diagnosis is based on typical ophthalmoscopic features. Fluorescein angiography reveals early mottled hyperfluorescence and late diffuse staining. Leakage from associated choroidal neovascularization may be seen.
- B-scan ultrasonography demonstrates a mildly elevated, highly reflective choroidal mass with acoustic shadowing.
- CT reveals focal hyperintensity similar to bone in the affected choroid.

PROGNOSIS AND MANAGEMENT

- Prognosis is variable. Visual loss may result from degeneration of the overlying RPE, choroidal neovascularization, or retinal detachment.
- Management consists of observation and, as appropriate, treatment of choroidal neovascularization.

FIGURE 6-15. **Choroidal osteoma.** Peripapillary choroidal osteoma is yellow-white in color and there are some overlying areas of clumping of brown pigment. B-scan ultrasonography of choroidal osteoma shows a highly reflective choroidal mass with acoustic shadowing behind the lesion; this is due to intrinsic bone. Courtesy of Drs. Jerry and Carol Shields, Oncology Service, Wills Eye Hospital, Philadelphia, Pennsylvania.

Congenital and Pediatric Retinal Diseases

Nikolas J.S. London and Richard S. Kaiser ▯

RETINOPATHY OF PREMATURITY

Retinopathy of prematurity (ROP) is a proliferative retinopathy of premature, low-birth-weight infants.

EPIDEMIOLOGY AND ETIOLOGY

- Despite recent advances, ROP remains a leading cause of visual loss in children. Infants born at less than 30 weeks gestation and/or those with a birth weight of 1500 g or less should be examined by indirect ophthalmoscopy. Infants who are born weighing 1000 g or less are at particularly high risk of developing severe ROP.

- The retinal vasculature of infants born prematurely has not completed its growth to the ora serrata. The developing vasculature is susceptible to capillary endothelial cytotoxicity. Pre-existing vessels are damaged and neovascularization develops off the surface of the retina. Continued growth and contraction of fibrovascular tissue may lead to retinal detachment.

HISTORY

- The critical components of the history are the birth weight, the gestational age at birth, the current postmenstrual age, and the current chronological age. One should also inquire regarding the use of mechanical ventilation and/or supplemental oxygen, the length of stay in the neonatal ICU, blood transfusions, the presence of any bronchodysplasia or hyaline membrane disease. Pregnancy history, maternal health, and family history are also often obtained.

DIAGNOSTIC EVALUATION

- Careful examination of neonates with indirect ophthalmoscopy in the intensive care nursery or at discharge is essential to detect ROP at a stage where treatment can be applied.

- Examinations should start at 31 weeks postmenstrual age or by 4 weeks chronological age, based on gestational age, and should continue every 1 to 3 weeks, until one of the following occurs:

- There is vascularization of zone III without prior zone I or II disease.
- Postmenstrual age 45 weeks is achieved with no prethreshold ROP.
- The retina is completely vascularized.
- There is total regression of treated ROP.

IMPORTANT CLINICAL SIGNS

- The posterior segment signs of ROP follow a progression of increasing severity that were classified according to the International Classification of ROP (ICROP).
- First the location of the disease is determined, then the stage of severity, and finally the extent of that stage is noted (**Table 7-1**, Figs. 7-1 to 7-5).

ASSOCIATED CLINICAL SIGNS

- "Plus" disease denotes increased severity. When an eye has dilation and tortuosity of the retinal vessels in the posterior pole, then it is said to have plus disease and has a poorer prognosis (Fig. 7-6). When vascularization is only present in zone I and there is plus disease, then a very poor prognosis exists because of the risk of rapid progression ("rush" disease).
- "Threshold" disease is a level of ROP at which it is predicted that there is a 50% chance of progression to retinal detachment without treatment. It was defined in the CRYO-ROP study as 5 contiguous clock hours of extraretinal fibrovascular proliferation (ERFP) with plus disease or 8 accumulated clock hours of ERFP with plus disease (Fig. 7-7). When threshold disease

TABLE 7-1. International Classification of Retinopathy of Prematurity (ICROP)

Location	
Zone I	Posterior circle of retina centered on the optic nerve with a radius of twice the disc-fovea distance
Zone II	Circular area of retina from the edge of zone I to the nasal ora serrata
Zone III	Remaining temporal crescent of retina
Extent	
Number of clock hours or 30-degree sectors involved	
Severity	
Stage 1	Demarcation line between posterior vascularized retina and anterior avascular retina
Stage 2	Demarcation line with height, width, and volume (ridge)
Stage 3	Ridge with extraretinal fibrovascular proliferation (ERFP); may be mild, moderate, or severe
Stage 4	Subtotal retinal detachment
4A	Extrafoveal
4B	Involving the fovea
Stage 5	Total retinal detachment; always funnel-shaped
	Open anteriorly, open posteriorly
	Open anteriorly, narrow posteriorly
	Narrow anteriorly, open posteriorly
	Narrow anteriorly, narrow posteriorly

is reached, treatment is recommended. In addition, current guidelines indicate treatment within 72 hours for the following clinical situations:

- Zone I, any stage, with plus disease

- Zone I, stage III, with or without plus disease

- Zone II, stage II or III, with plus disease

• Occasionally neovascular tissue may form buds of vascular proliferation behind the ridge or demarcation line. These lesions are called "popcorn" because of their similarity to popped corn (see Fig. 7-3A). These lesions do not carry any prognostic significance unless they are a part of ERFP at the advancing border of vascularization. Vitreous hemorrhage and preretinal hemorrhage can occasionally be seen in eyes with severe ERFP.

• In early cicatricial ROP (after resolution of the acute phase) there may be a variety of tractional complications. A hallmark finding of regressed cicatricial ROP is temporal retinal dragging (Fig. 7-8).

• After regression of ROP, either spontaneously or with treatment, several associated abnormalities may occur.

- Myopia
- Astigmatism
- Strabismus
- Amblyopia
- Cataract
- Glaucoma
- Macular ectopia
- Retinal fold
- Retinal detachment—rhegmatogenous or exudative

DIFFERENTIAL DIAGNOSIS

• The clinical setting usually aids in the diagnosis of ROP. Infants are born prematurely and are of low birth weight with a history of oxygen exposure.

• Differential diagnosis depends on the stage of the disease. In less severe ROP, conditions that cause peripheral retinal vascular changes and retinal dragging should be considered.

- Familial exudative vitreoretinopathy (FEVR)
- Incontinentia pigmenti (Bloch–Sulzberger syndrome)
- X-linked retinoschisis
- Norrie's disease

• In advanced cicatricial ROP, the differential diagnosis is that of retinal detachment or a white pupillary reflex, or both.

- Cataract
- FEVR
- Persistent fetal vasculature (PFV)
- Ocular toxocariasis
- Intermediate uveitis
- Coats' disease
- Retinoblastoma
- Vitreous hemorrhage
- Retinal detachment
- Endophthalmitis

PROGNOSIS AND MANAGEMENT

• The majority of infants who develop ROP undergo spontaneous regression (85%). However, 7% of infants weighing less than 1251 g at birth will develop threshold ROP.

• Cryotherapy to the anterior avascular zone (Fig. 7-9) has been shown to reduce the likelihood of an unfavorable outcome (retinal fold through zone I, retinal detachment, or retrolental fibroplasia) by 50% in the cryotherapy for ROP Study. Visual results are commensurately improved.

• Laser photocoagulation delivered with an indirect ophthalmoscope to the anterior avascular zone has virtually replaced cryotherapy for threshold ROP (Fig. 7-10). Laser burns should be spaced evenly, approximately one-half burn width apart, with particular attention to the most posterior avascular retina. Better visual outcomes have been achieved with laser treatment.

• Antiangiogenic injection therapy for ROP is being investigated, with early reports of success. Bevacizumab eliminates the angiogenic threat of ROP is a randomized trial comparing intravitreal bevacizumab to conventional laser treatment.

• More advanced stages of ROP (stages 4 and 5 retinal detachment) can be treated with scleral buckling or vitrectomy, or both. The prognosis for visual recovery after retinal detachment remains poor.

FIGURE 7-1. Retinopathy of prematurity (ROP). Schematic diagram of division of fundus into zones for defining location of involvement with ROP.

FIGURE 7-2. ROP, stage 2. The demarcation line (*arrow*) between posterior vascularized and anterior avascular retina is elevated as a ridge.

FIGURE 7-3. ROP, stage 3. A. The ridge has fibrovascular tissue and is elevated off the surface of the retina (extraretinal fibrovascular proliferation, or ERFP). This is an example of severe stage 3 ROP. Buds of vascular proliferation behind the ridge are "popcorn" lesions (*arrow*). **B.** Fluorescein angiogram from same patient as in **A** showing intense hyperfluorescence from vascular proliferative tissue in region of ridge.

FIGURE 7-4. ROP, stage 5. Eye with shallow total retinal detachment. Note loss of choroidal detail due to shallow subretinal fluid accumulation in posterior pole.

FIGURE 7-5. ROP, stage 5. This eye has a total tractional retinal detachment due to severe fibrous proliferation with contraction of the fibrous tissue. Note the vascularized tissue behind the clear lens.

FIGURE 7-6. ROP, plus disease. Dilation and tortuosity of vessels in the posterior pole denotes progressive disease and is known as "plus" disease.

FIGURE 7-7. ROP, threshold disease. Schematic diagram of threshold disease according to the Cryotherapy for Retinopathy of Prematurity Study Group. Reprinted by permission of American Medical Association from Cryotherapy for Retinopathy of Prematurity Cooperative Group. Multicenter trial of cryotherapy of retinopathy of prematurity: Preliminary results. *Arch Ophthalmol* 1988;106:474.

FIGURE 7-8. **ROP.** Severe dragging of the temporal retina with vascular straightening (*arrow*) is a late cicatricial complication of ROP. Compare with familial exudative vitreoretinopathy, in Figure 7-18A.

FIGURE 7-9. ROP, cryotherapy. A. The arrow points to the anterior avascular zone where cryotherapy will be placed for threshold ROP. **B.** Late postoperative appearance of cryotherapy. Note regression of extraretinal fibrovascular proliferation.

FIGURE 7-10. ROP. A. Preoperative appearance of an eye with posterior threshold ROP. **B.** Late postoperative appearance after laser photocoagulation. Note regression of extraretinal fibrovascular proliferation.

INCONTINENTIA PIGMENTI

Incontinentia pigmenti, or Bloch–Sulzberger syndrome, is a rare X-linked dominant condition that includes ocular, skin, central nervous system, skeletal, dental, and other systemic abnormalities.

EPIDEMIOLOGY AND ETIOLOGY

- The pathogenesis of incontinentia pigmenti is unknown. It is an X-linked dominant condition that is usually lethal in males and thus usually only seen in female infants. However, an affected male with Klinefelter syndrome (XXY) or a genetic mosaicism may survive.

HISTORY

- Characteristic skin changes usually start days after birth, with ophthalmic findings developing in infancy or even later in life.

IMPORTANT CLINICAL SIGNS

- Approximately one-third of infants with incontinentia pigmenti have ocular findings. Fundus abnormalities include dilated, tortuous retinal vessels, peripheral retinal capillary nonperfusion with arteriovenous anastomoses and neovascularization (Figs. 7-11 and 7-12), foveal hypoplasia, branch artery occlusions, neovascularization of the disc, retinal dragging, tractional and rhegmatogenous retinal detachments, retinal folds, vitreous hemorrhage, and optic disc pallor.

- The ocular abnormalities are often extremely asymmetric.

ASSOCIATED CLINICAL SIGNS

- Other ocular findings include cataract, conjunctival pigmentation, and strabismus. Skin findings, for which the disease is named, include vesicular skin eruptions (Fig. 7-13) that later turn into depigmented lesions (Fig. 7-14). These changes start days after birth.

- Dental abnormalities consisting of missing or cone-shaped teeth are present in approximately two-thirds of affected individuals (Fig. 7-15). Associated central nervous system abnormalities include seizures, spastic paralysis, and mental retardation.

DIFFERENTIAL DIAGNOSIS

- As for early stages of ROP:
  - FEVR
  - Incontinentia pigmenti (Bloch–Sulzberger syndrome)
  - X-linked retinoschisis
  - Norrie's disease
- If retinal detachment is a presenting finding, other causes of infantile retinal detachment should be considered.

DIAGNOSTIC EVALUATION

- Clinical evaluation including examination of the skin may lead to a diagnosis of incontinentia pigmenti.

PROGNOSIS AND MANAGEMENT

- Most patients with incontinentia pigmenti require no treatment.

- Progressive peripheral retinal neovascularization may respond to laser photocoagulation or cryotherapy. Intravitreal anti-VEGF agents have been used with limited success.

- Retinal detachments may be repaired with scleral buckling or vitrectomy, or both.

FIGURE 7-11. **Incontinentia pigmenti.** Peripheral fundus of a patient with incontinentia pigmenti showing peripheral retinal capillary nonperfusion and arteriovenous anastomoses (*arrow*).

FIGURE 7-12. **Incontinentia pigmenti.** Fluorescein angiogram of the peripheral fundus of a patient with incontinentia pigmenti showing peripheral retinal capillary nonperfusion and arteriovenous anastomoses (*arrow*).

FIGURE 7-13. **Incontinentia pigmenti, dermatologic findings.** Vesicular skin lesions in an infant with incontinentia pigmenti.

FIGURE 7-14. **Incontinentia pigmenti, dermatologic findings.** Pigmentary alteration of the skin in a patient with resolved vesicular eruptions of incontinentia pigmenti.

FIGURE 7-15. Incontinentia pigmenti, dental findings. Dental x-ray of cone-shaped tooth in a patient with incontinentia pigmenti.

FAMILIAL EXUDATIVE VITREORETINOPATHY

- FEVR is a group of autosomal-dominant fundus disorders characterized by peripheral retinal nonperfusion and neovascularization.

EPIDEMIOLOGY AND ETIOLOGY

- The exact etiology of FEVR is unknown. It is an autosomal-dominant hereditary disorder (rare cases of X-linked inheritance have been reported) that is asymptomatic in 50% of cases.

HISTORY

- Infants born with FEVR are otherwise healthy. There is usually no history of prematurity, oxygen exposure, or respiratory difficulties.
- The clinical features vary considerably and, although bilateral, there is often asymmetry.
- Infants may present with strabismus or a white pupillary reflex if the findings are severe. However, symptoms of decreased vision may occur at any age.

IMPORTANT CLINICAL SIGNS

- The classic finding in FEVR is peripheral retinal capillary nonperfusion (Fig. 7-16). Peripheral neovascularization may form at the border of posterior vascularized and anterior avascular retina (Fig. 7-17). Retinal dragging from contraction of fibrovascular tissue may occur (Fig. 7-18). Vitreous hemorrhage rarely occurs.

- Progression to more severe changes such as tractional, exudative, and even rhegmatogenous retinal detachment may occur (Fig. 7-19). Intraretinal and subretinal lipid exudation may sometimes occur.
- The findings are often asymmetric.

ASSOCIATED CLINICAL SIGNS

- In severe cases with retinal detachment, there may be cataract, band keratopathy, neovascular glaucoma, phthisis, or a combination of these findings.

DIFFERENTIAL DIAGNOSIS

- As for early stages of ROP:
  - FEVR
  - Incontinentia pigmenti (Bloch–Sulzberger syndrome)
  - X-linked retinoschisis
  - Norrie's disease
- If retinal detachment is a presenting finding, other causes of infantile retinal detachment should be considered.

DIAGNOSTIC EVALUATION

- Typical fundus findings are noted on ophthalmoscopy.
- If FEVR is suspected, examination of the peripheral retina of asymptomatic family members may reveal findings consistent with the diagnosis.

PROGNOSIS AND MANAGEMENT

- Patients who are affected at a young age usually have more severe pathology. Laser photocoagulation or cryotherapy to the peripheral avascular retina may prevent progression of fibrovascular complications.

- Scleral buckling and vitrectomy surgery have been attempted for more severe cases with retinal detachment.

- All family members of an affected individual should be examined, because progressive changes may occur throughout life.

FIGURE 7-16. **Familial exudative vitreoretinopathy (FEVR).** Peripheral retinal capillary nonperfusion (*arrow*) in FEVR appears featureless.

FIGURE 7-17. FEVR. A. Clinical photograph showing peripheral retinal capillary nonperfusion with some intraretinal lipid exudate (*arrow*). **B.** Corresponding fluorescein angiogram documenting peripheral nonperfusion and areas of neovascularization.

FIGURE 7-18. FEVR. A. Temporal dragging of the retina with vascular straightening (*arrow*). Compare with ROP, Figure 7-8. **B.** Temporal periphery with intraretinal lipid, peripheral retinal capillary nonperfusion, and peripheral neovascularization (*arrow*).

FIGURE 7-19. **FEVR.** Severe tractional retinal detachment with dragging.

COATS' DISEASE

Coats' disease is a unilateral, idiopathic retinal vascular abnormality first described by George Coats in 1908. It is characterized by telangiectatic retinal vascular abnormalities in association with lipid exudation. Coats' disease should be differentiated from a *Coats' response,* or a large degree of lipid exudation, which can occur with abnormalities such as retinitis pigmentosa, diabetic retinopathy, retinal venous obstruction, retinal capillary hemangioma, and the late sequelae of ROP.

EPIDEMIOLOGY AND ETIOLOGY

• Coats' disease is idiopathic. Most cases are diagnosed before age 20 with the peak incidence at the end of the first decade.
• It occurs predominately in males (85%) and is almost always uniocular.
• The severity of the disease varies widely from asymptomatic patches of telangiectatic vessels in the retinal periphery (Fig. 7-20) to total exudative retinal detachment (Fig. 7-21).

HISTORY

• Infants may present with strabismus, leukokoria, or a red, painful eye (from neovascular glaucoma).
• The severity and rate of progression are greatest in younger patients (less than 4 years of age).
• Older children and, rarely, adults may complain of reduced vision in one eye.

PATHOPHYSIOLOGY

• The retinal vessels become telangiectatic and develop multiple aneurysmal abnormalities. These can occur on the retinal arterial or venous sides, or both.
• Marked hard exudation is frequently present, extending from the retina into the subretinal space when it is massive.

IMPORTANT CLINICAL SIGNS

• Telangiectatic vessels, venous dilation, microaneurysms, and fusiform capillary dilation are the hallmark findings of Coats' disease (Fig. 7-22).
• Progressive exudation from these retinal vascular abnormalities may lead to exudative retinal detachment.

ASSOCIATED CLINICAL SIGNS

• Posterior segment neovascularization is rare even though retinal capillary nonperfusion is often present. Retinal telangiectasis has been reported in association with many other ocular and systemic diseases. Retinitis pigmentosa with a "Coats'-like response" has been documented.
• Other entities associated with retinal telangiectasia are Alport's syndrome, tuberous sclerosis, Turner's syndrome, Senior–Loken syndrome, the ichthyosis hystrix variant of epidermal nevus syndrome, muscular dystrophy, and fascio-scaspulohumeral dystrophy.

DIFFERENTIAL DIAGNOSIS

• The differential diagnosis of Coats' disease depends on the severity of the disease being considered.
• Childhood disease (leukokoria or exudative retinal detachment)
  ▪ Retinoblastoma

- Persistent hyperplastic primary vitreous (PHPV)/PFV
- ROP
- FEVR
- Norrie's disease
- Ocular toxocariasis
- Von Hippel–Lindau disease
- Peripheral exudative vitreoretinopathy
- Incontinentia pigmenti (Bloch–Sulzberger syndrome)
- Pars planitis
- Retinitis pigmentosa with Coats'-like response
- Vitreous hemorrhage
- Parafoveal telangiectasia with or without lipid exudation
  - Diabetic retinopathy
  - Radiation retinopathy
  - Juxtafoveal retinal telangiectasia
  - Branch retinal vein occlusion
- Localized telangiectasia with arterial or venous aneurysms
  - Retinal cavernous hemangioma
  - Acquired retinal arterial macroaneurysm
  - Idiopathic retinal vasculitis, aneurysms, and neuroretinitis (IRVAN)

DIAGNOSTIC EVALUATION

- The diagnosis is usually made through ophthalmoscopy; however, fluorescein angiography may be helpful in detecting telangiectatic retinal vascular abnormalities. Characteristic "lightbulb" aneurysmal dilations of larger retinal vessels are particularly obvious on fluorescein angiography (Fig. 7-23). Retinal capillary nonperfusion may also be seen with fluorescein angiography.

- In cases with a poor view of the fundus, ultrasonography is helpful and may exhibit a hyperechoic mass in the posterior vitreous, occasionally with evidence of vitreous and/or subretinal hemorrhage.

PROGNOSIS AND MANAGEMENT

- Management consists of observation; cryotherapy or laser photocoagulation may be applied to areas of retinal vascular abnormalities with progressive exudation (Fig. 7-24). Multiple treatment sessions are often necessary and close follow-up is warranted because recurrences have been reported up to 5 years after complete resolution.

- Vitrectomy and scleral buckling can be considered for retinal detachment, total retinal detachment typically results in permanent, profound vision loss despite intervention.

- Enucleation should be considered for eyes with no light perception and persistent pain.

FIGURE 7-20. Coats' disease. A. Peripheral fundus of an asymptomatic patient with microaneurysms, intraretinal hemorrhages, and lipid exudates. **B.** Posterior pole of the same patient with a normal macula.

FIGURE 7-21. **Coats' disease.** Total exudative retinal detachment.

FIGURE 7-22. **Coats' disease.** Peripheral fundus demonstrating venous dilation, microaneurysms, subretinal lipid exudation (*arrow*), and larger retinal vessels with "lightbulb" aneurysmal dilations (inset).

FIGURE 7-23. Coats' disease. Fluorescein angiogram of the same patient as in Figure 7-22 clearly showing dilated retinal vessels with aneurysmal dilations.

FIGURE 7-24. **Coats' disease. A.** Peripheral fundus showing aneurysmal dilation and hemorrhage with some exudation from Coats' disease. **B.** Same area 4 months after cryotherapy showing involution of aneurysms and resolution of hemorrhage and exudates.

CHORIORETINAL COLOBOMA

A chorioretinal coloboma is a developmental abnormality caused by failure of complete closure of the embryonic fissure.

EPIDEMIOLOGY AND ETIOLOGY

- Chorioretinal coloboma is a congenital developmental abnormality. There are rare cases of autosomal-recessive inheritance.
- The retina and choroid are absent in areas affected. A thin intercalary membrane covers the sclera. This membrane consists of rudimentary retina with blood vessels. The coloboma is located inferiorly, because the embryonic fissure is located inferonasally in the developing eye.

HISTORY

- Patients are usually asymptomatic unless the optic nerve or macula are involved or if there are secondary effects.
- Retinal breaks may occur in the intercalary membrane. Retinal detachment may then occur and cause symptoms.

IMPORTANT CLINICAL SIGNS

- A white area (sclera) is visible in the inferior fundus to a variable extent depending on the size of the defect (Fig. 7-25).
- The margins of the coloboma are well defined.

- There is often a pigmented border marking the transition from the coloboma to the normal retina and choroid.

ASSOCIATED CLINICAL SIGNS

- The coloboma may extend back to the optic nerve (Fig. 7-26) and forward to involve the ciliary body, zonules, and iris.
- The lens may be flattened at the pole corresponding to the coloboma owing to the missing zonule (Fig. 7-27).

DIFFERENTIAL DIAGNOSIS

- Chorioretinal scar (e.g., ocular toxoplasmosis)
- Degenerative myopia

DIAGNOSTIC EVALUATION

- Ophthalmoscopy usually suffices to make the diagnosis of chorioretinal coloboma.

PROGNOSIS AND MANAGEMENT

- No treatment is necessary unless retinal detachment occurs (Fig. 7-28).
- Vitrectomy surgery is necessary to manage the retinal detachment associated with chorioretinal coloboma. Internal drainage through the hole in the intercalary membrane is performed (if the hole can be found) and laser photocoagulation is placed around the margins of the coloboma.

FIGURE 7-25. **Chorioretinal coloboma.** Chorioretinal defect in the inferior fundus.

FIGURE 7-26. **Chorioretinal coloboma.** Colobomatous defect involving the inferior fundus and optic nerve.

FIGURE 7-27. **Chorioretinal coloboma.** Extension of coloboma anteriorly. Note flattening of the inferior pole of the lens (*arrow*) due to the missing portion of the zonule.

FIGURE 7-28. Chorioretinal coloboma. Posterior pole (**A**) and inferonasal area (**B**) of a patient with chorioretinal coloboma and associated rhegmatogenous retinal detachment.

PERSISTENT HYPERPLASTIC PRIMARY VITREOUS/PERSISTENT FETAL VASCULATURE

PHPV was thought to be caused by failure of the primary vitreous to regress. Now the term PFV has been proposed to integrate the findings that occur when there is failure of regression of components of the fetal vessels.

EPIDEMIOLOGY AND ETIOLOGY

- PFV is a rare developmental abnormality.
- The condition is almost always unilateral and is more common in males than females.
- Anterior and posterior forms exist, and both may be present together.

HISTORY

- In the anterior form, infants present with leukokoria due to a white, vascularized fibrous membrane behind the lens.
- In the posterior form, the eye may be microphthalmic but the anterior segment is otherwise normal. The infant may present with leukokoria due to a persistent stalk of tissue from the optic nerve to the retrolental region.

IMPORTANT CLINICAL SIGNS

- In the anterior form, microphthalmia, a shallow anterior chamber and long ciliary processes visible through the pupil are seen in association with the white pupillary reflex (Fig. 7-29).
- In the posterior form, the eye may be microphthalmic with a clear lens and no retrolental membrane. There is a stalk of tissue emanating from the optic disc to the retrolental area (Fig. 7-30).
- Often, an associated retinal fold is located in an inferior quadrant.

ASSOCIATED CLINICAL SIGNS

- Cataract and narrow-angle glaucoma may occur in the anterior form of PFV if a dehiscence in the lens capsule occurs.
- Severe cases may progress to retinal detachment and phthisis bulbi.

DIFFERENTIAL DIAGNOSIS

- The differential diagnosis of the anterior PFV is that of leukokoria.
- The differential diagnosis of the posterior PFV is ROP, ocular toxocariasis, and FEVR.

DIAGNOSTIC EVALUATION

- Clinical examination of the anterior segment is important in establishing the diagnosis of PFV. If the anterior segment is not affected, the diagnosis of the posterior PFV can be established by ophthalmoscopy.
- Ultrasonography and computed tomographic (CT) scanning may help differentiate PFV from retinoblastoma, especially when the anterior segment is involved.

PROGNOSIS AND MANAGEMENT

- Pars plana vitrectomy, lensectomy removal of the fibrovascular retrolental membrane, and anterior vitrectomy in the anterior PFV help prevent narrow-angle glaucoma, but visual results are poor.

FIGURE 7-29. Persistent hyperplastic primary vitreous (PHPV)/persistent fetal vasculature (PFV).
Anterior PHPV/PFV in a microphthalmic eye. Note the white reflex due to vascularized membrane behind the lens and ciliary processes dragged in toward the center.

FIGURE 7-30. PHPV/PFV. External view of posterior PHPV/PFV. Note termination of the stalk of tissue on the posterior surface of the lens. Ciliary processes are not dragged in toward the center.

JUVENILE X-LINKED RETINOSCHISIS

Juvenile X-linked retinoschisis is a hereditary disorder characterized by diffuse retinal dysfunction with a stellate macula in all cases and splitting of the nerve fiber layer in 50% of cases.

EPIDEMIOLOGY AND ETIOLOGY

- Juvenile X-linked retinoschisis is a bilateral inherited disorder occurring in males. Linkage studies have localized the retinoschisis gene to the distal short arm of the X chromosome (Xp22.1–p22.3).
- The electroretinographic abnormalities implicate Müller cell dysfunction.

HISTORY

- Patients may present with reduced vision from the macular changes.
- Earlier presentation occurs due to routine examination of family members with a family history of the disease.
- In patients with severe peripheral involvement, vitreous hemorrhage resulting from rupture of unsupported retinal vessels in the elevated nerve fiber layer may cause abrupt loss of vision.

IMPORTANT CLINICAL SIGNS

- Foveal schisis is present in all cases and appears as a stellate maculopathy on ophthalmoscopic examination (Fig. 7-31). The stellate appearance often gives way to ill-defined retinal pigment epithelial alterations in older patients.
- Peripheral retinoschisis is present in 50% of patients (Fig. 7-32). It is most common inferiorly and is at the level of the nerve fiber layer. Often, breaks occur in the elevated nerve fiber layer leaving unsupported retinal vessels that can rupture, causing vitreous hemorrhage (Fig. 7-33). Breaks can occur in the inner layer causing rhegmatogenous retinal detachment (Fig. 7-34).

ASSOCIATED CLINICAL SIGNS

- Less common findings include traction or exudative retinal detachment, extension of the retinoschisis into the macula, macular ectopia with nasal or temporal dragging, hypermetropia, cataract, and strabismus.

DIFFERENTIAL DIAGNOSIS

- ROP
- Goldmann–Favre disease
- Retinitis pigmentosa
- FEVR

DIAGNOSTIC EVALUATION

- The stellate macula is often best seen with red-free illumination. Although it has the appearance of cystoid macular edema, there is no leakage of dye on fluorescein angiography.
- Electroretinography is useful because patients typically have selective loss of the b-wave.
- Examination of family members, some of whom may have the disease, may aid in diagnosis.

PROGNOSIS AND MANAGEMENT

- There is no treatment for the macular aspects of the disease.
- Vitrectomy can be performed for non-clearing vitreous hemorrhage.
- Retinal detachment repair can be attempted with scleral buckling or vitrectomy techniques.
- Genetic counseling should be offered.

FIGURE 7-31. Juvenile X-linked retinoschisis. A. Foveal schisis. **B.** High-power image of foveal schisis; note radiating retinal striae.

FIGURE 7-32. **Juvenile X-linked retinoschisis.** Highly bullous peripheral retinoschisis.

FIGURE 7-33. Juvenile X-linked retinoschisis. Inferior retinoschisis with large breaks (*arrow*) and unsupported retinal vessels (*).

FIGURE 7-34. Juvenile X-linked retinoschisis. Rhegmatogenous retinal detachment in a patient with juvenile X-linked retinoschisis. Note the stellate appearance in the macula due to foveal schisis.

LEBER'S CONGENITAL AMAUROSIS

Leber's congenital amaurosis is a group of diseases characterized by severe loss of vision from birth associated with nystagmus and severely impaired electroretinogram (ERG) responses for both rods and cones.

EPIDEMIOLOGY AND ETIOLOGY

- Leber's congenital amaurosis is a hereditary disease most commonly inherited as an autosomal-recessive trait.
- Several genetic defects have been identified.

HISTORY

- Patients usually present because of nystagmus or strabismus; however, parents may be concerned earlier that the infant does not recognize faces.

IMPORTANT CLINICAL SIGNS

- The fundi are usually normal. Horizontal nystagmus is present.

ASSOCIATED CLINICAL SIGNS

- Many children are highly hyperopic.
- Older children may develop cataracts and keratoconus.

DIFFERENTIAL DIAGNOSIS

- Albinism
- Congenital stationary night blindness
- Achromatopsia

DIAGNOSTIC EVALUATION

- Fundus examination is often not helpful because infants may have a normal-appearing fundus. Arteriolar attenuation, optic nerve pallor, and pigmentary degeneration may occur later in childhood (Fig. 7-35).
- Electrophysiologic testing is necessary to establish a diagnosis. The ERG is typically minimal or extinguished.

PROGNOSIS AND MANAGEMENT

- There is no treatment available.

FIGURE 7-35. Leber's congenital amaurosis. Fundus of an older child demonstrating one of the late patterns of Leber's congenital amaurosis. Note pigmentary retinopathy and "macular coloboma," chorioretinal degeneration in the macula.

Traumatic and Toxic Retinopathies

J. Luigi Borrillo and Carl D. Regillo ▮

COMMOTIO RETINAE

Commotio retinae is retinal whitening that occurs after blunt ocular trauma. This transient condition affects the outer retina. Often the damage incurred to the photoreceptors is reversible.

EPIDEMIOLOGY

• Statistically the condition is most common in young males.

HISTORY

• Patients have a history of blunt ocular trauma.

CLINICAL SIGNS

• The condition is usually asymptomatic. Decreased vision may occur with macular involvement. The retina appears whitened, while the retinal vasculature remains unaffected. The retina regains its normal appearance within weeks (Fig. 8-1). Occasionally, changes to the retinal pigment epithelium (RPE), such as stippling or clumping, may be seen after the retinal whitening resolves.

• Be mindful of other findings seen in trauma such as hyphema or microhyphema, choroidal rupture, retinal hemorrhage, retinal dialysis, avulsed vitreous base, and vitreous hemorrhage.

DIFFERENTIAL DIAGNOSIS

• Other entities that may mimic commotio retinae include branch retinal artery occlusion, white-without-pressure, and shallow retinal detachment.

DIAGNOSTIC EVALUATION

• Diagnosis is based on clinical examination.

• Optical coherence tomography (OCT) may demonstrate increased reflectivity in areas of damaged photoreceptor outer segments.

PROGNOSIS AND MANAGEMENT

• Retinal whitening resolves without visual compromise. However, permanent visual acuity loss can sometimes occur if macular retinal pigment epithelial disruption is present.

FIGURE 8-1. Commotio retinae. A. Commotio retinae: Outer retinal whitening in the posterior pole after blunt trauma. **B.** Outer retinal whitening in the peripheral retina.

CHOROIDAL RUPTURE

In this injury, disruption of the choriocapillaris and Bruch's membrane occurs secondary to traumatic ocular compression. Ruptures located in the posterior pole are concentric to the optic disc. These breaks are often associated with subretinal and subretinal pigment epithelial hemorrhage.

EPIDEMIOLOGY AND ETIOLOGY

- Choroidal rupture occurs as a result of trauma, most commonly in young males.

HISTORY

- Patients have a history of blunt ocular trauma.

CLINICAL SIGNS

- The characteristic finding is subretinal hemorrhage, with whitish, crescent-shaped lesions around the optic disc (Fig. 8-2A). In the acute setting, choroidal ruptures may be associated with other findings from blunt ocular trauma such as hyphema, iris sphincter ruptures, commotio retinae, vitreous hemorrhage, retinal tears, retinal dialysis, and orbital fractures.

- Later, choroidal neovascularization (CNV) may occur at the edge of the rupture site (Fig. 8-2B).

DIFFERENTIAL DIAGNOSIS

- Myopic lacquer cracks and angioid streaks may have a similar appearance.

- Other causes of subretinal hemorrhage include CNV, retinal arterial macroaneurysm, Valsalva retinopathy, and anemia.

DIAGNOSTIC EVALUATION

- Diagnosis is based on clinical examination.

PROGNOSIS AND MANAGEMENT

- Visual prognosis depends on the location of the choroidal rupture with respect to the fovea and any associated subretinal or subretinal pigment epithelial hemorrhage.

- Secondary CNV can occur at anytime during the follow-up period and can cause visual acuity loss.

FIGURE 8-2. Choroidal rupture. A. Choroidal rupture: Crescent-shaped lesion in the macula with subretinal hemorrhage (inset). **B.** Chronic choroidal rupture: Yellow crescent-shaped rupture site with pigmented choroidal neovascularization (*arrow*) and associated subretinal fluid in the fovea.

AVULSED VITREOUS BASE

This entity describes separation of the vitreous base at the ora serrata that occurs secondary to trauma. Sometimes the avulsed vitreous base can be seen floating in the periphery.

EPIDEMIOLOGY AND ETIOLOGY

- The injury occurs as a result of trauma, usually in young males.

HISTORY

- Patients have a history of blunt ocular trauma.

CLINICAL SIGNS

- A semitransparent, sometimes pigmented, curvilinear ribbon-like structure may or may not be completely separated from the retinal periphery (Fig. 8-3).
- The presence of an avulsed vitreous base is pathognomonic for ocular trauma.

- An avulsed vitreous base may be associated with hyphema, iris sphincter tears, commotio retinae, vitreous hemorrhage, retinal tears, retinal dialysis, or orbital fractures.

DIFFERENTIAL DIAGNOSIS

- Avulsed vitreous base should be distinguished from retinal dialysis.
- Other entities that may mimic this condition include old vitreous hemorrhage.

DIAGNOSTIC EVALUATION

- Diagnosis is based on binocular indirect ophthalmoscopy with scleral depression.

PROGNOSIS AND MANAGEMENT

- No treatment is necessary. Patients should be observed for the subsequent development of trauma-related ocular problems such as retinal breaks and angle-recession glaucoma.

FIGURE 8-3. **Avulsed vitreous base.** Nasal avulsed vitreous base (*arrow*) is pathognomonic for prior trauma.

SOLAR MACULOPATHY

Solar maculopathy is the visual loss resulting from foveal photoreceptor and retinal pigment epithelial damage as a consequence of sungazing or direct observation of a solar eclipse.

EPIDEMIOLOGY

• There is a trend for higher incidence in areas where a solar eclipse was directly observable. Solar maculopathy is more common among individuals involved in sunworshiping religious groups. Loss of the ozone layer has been associated with solar retinopathy among sunbathers in the United States.

HISTORY

• Patients have a history of sungazing.

CLINICAL SIGNS

• There is an abnormal foveal reflex.

• Often, a sharply demarcated yellow or reddish spot is visible in the fovea (**Fig. 8-4**).

• Retinal pigment epithelial changes (focal hyperpigmentation) may be evident in the foveal or parafoveal area at later stages.

DIFFERENTIAL DIAGNOSIS

• Pseudomacular hole, photic maculopathy, and macular dystrophy or degeneration may have a similar appearance.

DIAGNOSTIC EVALUATION

• Diagnosis is based on clinical examination.

• Fluorescein angiography will reveal nonspecific retinal pigment epithelial window defects centered on the fovea.

• OCT may demonstrate disruption of foveal inner and outer photoreceptor segments.

PROGNOSIS AND MANAGEMENT

• Good visual recovery occurs in most patients, but it may take weeks or months for vision to improve.

• No treatment is needed.

FIGURE 8-4. Solar retinopathy. A. Color fundus photograph demonstrating deep yellow foveal lesion (inset).

(*continued*)

FIGURE 8-4. (*Continued*) **Solar retinopathy. B.** Corresponding fluorescein angiogram photograph demonstrating foveal window defect. **C.** Acute solar retinopathy with yellow foveal lesion and hemorrhage. Visual acuity is 20/30. (**B,** Courtesy of Dr. Alexander J. Brucker.)

VALSALVA RETINOPATHY

In Valsalva retinopathy, unilateral or bilateral retinal or preretinal hemorrhage occurs as a result of an acute episode of increased intrathoracic pressure. Superficial capillaries rupture secondary to a sharp rise in ocular intravenous pressure.

EPIDEMIOLOGY

● The condition can occur in persons of any age.

HISTORY

● Patients usually have a history of recent strenuous physical exertion, coughing, vomiting, or straining (e.g., with constipation).

CLINICAL SIGNS

● Single or multiple intraretinal hemorrhages (often underneath the internal limiting membrane) are noted in the posterior pole (**Fig. 8-5**). There may be a decrease in visual acuity when the hemorrhage is localized in or over the foveal region.

● Subconjunctival hemorrhage may be associated with this condition. Significant vitreous hemorrhage is rare.

DIFFERENTIAL DIAGNOSIS

● Retinal macroaneurysm, diabetic retinopathy, venous occlusion, anemia, anticoagulant therapy, retinal tear, or posterior vitreous detachment with associated hemorrhage may mimic the findings of Valsalva retinopathy.

DIAGNOSTIC EVALUATION

● Diagnosis is based on clinical examination.

● B-scan ultrasonography is performed to evaluate for underlying retinal detachment or retinal tear in the setting of dense vitreous hemorrhage.

● OCT may demonstrate hemorrhage underneath reflective signal of the internal limiting membrane.

PROGNOSIS AND MANAGEMENT

● The visual prognosis is good.

● Management consists of observation, only, in most cases. Hemorrhages will resolve spontaneously.

● Vitrectomy may be considered for non-clearing vitreous hemorrhage (but is rarely indicated).

FIGURE 8-5. **Valsalva retinopathy.** Multiple superficial retinal hemorrhages in the macula.

SHAKEN BABY SYNDROME

This condition refers to intraocular hemorrhages in infants or young children secondary to child abuse. The findings are associated with decreased visual acuity and increased mortality.

EPIDEMIOLOGY

- The condition is most common in infants and toddlers.

HISTORY

- Recently, often multiple episodes of violent shaking of the infant precede findings, although it is often difficult to obtain a history of abuse from the caretaker. Caretakers may refuse diagnostic evaluation.

CLINICAL SIGNS

- Subretinal, intraretinal, or preretinal hemorrhages are noted in one or (more commonly) both eyes (Fig. 8-6A). The preretinal hemorrhages are typically globular as opposed to flat (Fig. 8-6B). Other signs include poor visual or pupillary response. No single ocular finding is pathognomonic.

- Ecchymosis, long bone and rib fractures, lethargy, or developmental delay are common associated findings. Often the child has physical findings that do not match the reported mechanism of the injuries.

DIFFERENTIAL DIAGNOSIS

- Birth trauma: Intraretinal hemorrhages may be seen in newborns, especially with the use of forceps in the delivery. These hemorrhages resolve over the course of weeks and are often not associated with neurologic sequelae.

- Leukemia and intraocular infections may also mimic the ocular findings of shaken baby syndrome.

DIAGNOSTIC EVALUATION

- Clinical examination: Evaluation for delayed neurologic development and systemic signs of child abuse

- Head CT to evaluate for intracranial hemorrhage

- Bone scan is more sensitive in detecting fractures and exposes the child to less radiation while providing a whole body skeletal survey. Bone scan findings may tailor subsequent x-ray studies.

- X-ray studies: Fractures at different stages of healing, leg fractures prior to bipedal ambulation (prior to 12 months of age), and posterior rib fractures are highly suspicious for child abuse.

- Optical coherence tomography: Preretinal hemorrhage, vitreoretinal traction, and hemorrhagic macular retinoschisis may be observed.

PROGNOSIS AND MANAGEMENT

- A pediatric consultation should be considered to evaluate for child abuse. The prognosis is largely dependent on associated brain injury. Poor pupillary response, poor visual acuity, and retinal hemorrhages have been associated with high infant mortality. Conversely, the presence of good visual acuity and normal pupillary reflexes are associated with a better prognosis.

FIGURE 8-6. Shaken baby syndrome. A. Multiple intraretinal and preretinal hemorrhages in the posterior pole. **B.** Note the globular nature (*arrows*) of the preretinal hemorrhage in shaken baby syndrome. (**A,** Courtesy of Dr. Richard Spaide.)

TERSON'S SYNDROME

Terson's syndrome encompasses any intra-ocular (usually preretinal or vitreous) hemorrhage associated with either trauma-induced or spontaneous acute intracranial bleeding.

EPIDEMIOLOGY AND ETIOLOGY

● The syndrome may affect individuals of any age.

● The sudden increase in intracranial pressure directly or indirectly ruptures the peripapillary capillaries.

HISTORY

● The presentation may include severe headache or known acute neurologic event.

CLINICAL SIGNS

● Patients may have varying degrees of decreased visual acuity and multiple, usually bilateral, retinal hemorrhages (Fig 8-7). Vitreous hemorrhage can also occur and may be dense.

● Other ocular signs associated with Terson's syndrome include cranial nerve palsies, late-appearing epiretinal membrane, or tractional retinal detachment.

● The intracranial hemorrhages are usually located in the subarachnoid space.

Spontaneous hemorrhages are a result of vascular abnormalities such as aneurysms, arteriovenous malformations, or fistulas.

DIFFERENTIAL DIAGNOSIS

● Posterior vitreous detachment with vitreous hemorrhage, retinal vein occlusion, retinal tear, proliferative diabetic retinopathy, Valsalva retinopathy, or retinal arterial macroaneurysm may mimic Terson's syndrome.

DIAGNOSTIC EVALUATION

● Neuroimaging is performed, using computed tomography (CT) or magnetic resonance imaging (MRI). B-scan ultrasonography is used to evaluate for retinal detachment or retinal tear in cases where vitreous hemorrhage precludes a view of the posterior segment. Optical coherence tomography findings may be similar to Valsalva retinopathy.

PROGNOSIS AND MANAGEMENT

● The visual prognosis is often good.

● There can be a high mortality rate depending on the location and severity of the intracranial hemorrhage.

● Neurosurgical consultation is recommended.

● In cases of bilateral vitreous hemorrhage or dense nonclearing vitreous hemorrhage, vitrectomy may be considered.

FIGURE 8-7. **Terson's syndrome. A.** Multiple retinal and preretinal hemorrhages in the posterior pole of a patient who has suffered an acute subarachnoid hemorrhage. **B.** More severe retinal hemorrhaging and vitreous hemorrhage in Terson's syndrome.

PURTSCHER'S RETINOPATHY

Purtscher's retinopathy describes decreased vision associated with intraretinal hemorrhages and patches of retinal whitening secondary to severe crushing injuries to the torso or head. The fundus findings are concentrated in the peripapillary area and may be unilateral or bilateral.

EPIDEMIOLOGY AND ETIOLOGY

- Persons of any age may be affected.
- Endothelial damage leads to intravascular coagulopathy and granulocytic aggregation with microemboli formation.

HISTORY

- There is a history of compressive trauma.

CLINICAL SIGNS

- Acutely, severe vision loss is noted in one or both eyes.
- Cotton-wool spots centered on the optic disc, hemorrhages, exudates, and retinal edema are often seen.
- Fundus findings resolve over several weeks (Fig. 8-8A).
- Optic atrophy may be a late finding.

DIFFERENTIAL DIAGNOSIS

- This condition should be distinguished from Purtscher's-like retinopathy, which has a similar fundus presentation associated with microemboli of various compositions from a wide spectrum of systemic conditions such as pancreatitis, amniotic fluid embolism, collagen vascular disease, thrombotic thrombocytopenic purpura, and long bone fractures (Fig. 8.8B).
- Central retinal artery and vein occlusion may also mimic the findings of Purtscher's retinopathy.

DIAGNOSTIC EVALUATION

- CT imaging of chest and long bones is performed, when indicated.
- Fluorescein angiography typically reveals areas of retinal ischemia.
- Optical coherence tomography reveals edema of the nerve fiber layer and subretinal fluid.

PROGNOSIS AND MANAGEMENT

- Permanent visual loss may occur in half of the affected patients. No treatment is available.

FIGURE 8-8. **Purtscher's retinopathy. A.** Multiple peripapillary cotton-wool spots centered around the optic disc in a patient with massive chest trauma. **B.** Multiple cotton-wool spots, hemorrhage, and macular infarction in a man with Still's disease.

TRAUMATIC MACULAR HOLE

This entity describes a full-thickness macular hole occurring after blunt ocular trauma.

EPIDEMIOLOGY AND ETIOLOGY

- Persons of any age may be affected.
- The foveal defect develops as a result of vitreous traction or contusion necrosis of the retina and may be a direct consequence of globe deformation.

HISTORY

- There is a history of recent blunt trauma or whiplash injury.

CLINICAL SIGNS

- A full-thickness macular hole with irregular border is seen on clinical examination. Macular pigmentary changes are often observed (Fig. 8-9), as well as a positive Watzke–Allen sign.
- Other associated signs may include submacular hemorrhage, choroidal rupture, commotio retinae, or vitreous hemorrhage.

- The presence of a posterior vitreous detachment is unlikely.

DIFFERENTIAL DIAGNOSIS

- Solar retinopathy
- Nontraumatic macular hole
- Pseudohole secondary to epiretinal membrane

DIAGNOSTIC EVALUATION

- Careful contact lens biomicroscopy is indicated.
- Fluorescein angiography may reveal a hyperfluorescent spot at the fovea corresponding to a retinal pigment epithelial defect.
- Optical coherence tomography will reveal full-thickness neurosensory retinal loss in the fovea.

PROGNOSIS AND MANAGEMENT

- The visual prognosis is variable.
- Spontaneous closure of traumatic macular holes in young patients has been reported in the literature but is rare.
- A recent series suggests that the macular hole surgery may be beneficial, with a reported visual acuity of 20/50 or better in 64% of patients.

FIGURE 8-9. Traumatic macular hole. A. Small, irregular full-thickness macular hole (inset) and associated macular retinal pigment epithelial clumping. **B.** Larger, irregular traumatic macular hole (inset) with marked retinal pigment epithelial alterations and a choroidal rupture (*arrow*) inferior to the optic disc.

CHORIORETINITIS SCLOPETARIA

Chorioretinitis sclopetaria is full-thickness disruption of the choroid and retina secondary to the concussive forces of a nonpenetrating high-velocity projectile.

EPIDEMIOLOGY AND ETIOLOGY

- The injury is most common in young males.

- Traveling at high speeds, the projectile creates shock waves that can rupture choroid and retina but leave sclera intact. The defects are subsequently replaced by fibrous tissue.

HISTORY

- Patients have a history of a high-velocity projectile, such as a BB pellet, to the orbit.

CLINICAL SIGNS

- The visual acuity is variable. Acutely, there may be preretinal, intraretinal, or subretinal hemorrhage as well as vitreous hemorrhage (**Fig. 8-10A**). Subsequently, lesions have a "claw-like" branching pattern (**Fig. 8-10B**). Bare sclera may be visible through the full-thickness defects of the choroid and overlying retina. Sclopetaria is usually located in the peripheral fundus, corresponding to the path of the projectile. Often these areas are covered by hemorrhage.

- Fibrous proliferation at the rupture sites eventually ensues and becomes visible as any associated hemorrhage clears. Intraorbital foreign body is often present.

DIFFERENTIAL DIAGNOSIS

- A ruptured globe should be ruled out.
- Choroidal ruptures may demonstrate a similar appearance as sclopetaria, but they are usually located in the posterior pole.

DIAGNOSTIC EVALUATION

- CT imaging is important to evaluate the integrity of the globe, detect any associated orbital or central nervous system injuries, and identify any orbital foreign bodies.

PROGNOSIS AND MANAGEMENT

- Visual prognosis is dependent on the location of sclopetaria. Lesions involving the macular region have poorer visual acuity.

- Initial management is nonsurgical. The subsequent cicatricial process often fuses tissues, making retinal detachments unlikely. Surgery is indicated in the subsequent development of retinal detachment or for the removal of nonclearing vitreous hemorrhage.

FIGURE 8-10. Chorioretinitis sclopetaria. A. Retinal whitening and preretinal hemorrhage in the posterior pole of a patient sustaining an orbital foreign body injury. **B.** Claw-like chorioretinal scarring after a high-velocity bullet passed through the orbit adjacent to the eye.

INTRAOCULAR FOREIGN BODY

Intraocular foreign body (IOFB) refers to the presence of a foreign body in the eye from a penetrating injury.

EPIDEMIOLOGY AND ETIOLOGY

- Young males are most commonly affected.
- The foreign body may serve as a nidus for endophthalmitis or severe inflammatory reaction.
- An IOFB may also cause delayed effects secondary to proliferative vitreoretinopathy or toxicity.

HISTORY

- Most often there is a history of penetrating ocular injury.
- A foreign body sensation associated with hammering, grinding, or other mechanism of injury may also be elicited. Injury in a rural setting increases the risk of secondary endophthalmitis.

CLINICAL SIGNS

- Visual acuity is variable. An obvious or subtle point of entry of the IOFB may be seen (Fig. 8-11A). Other signs associated with IOFBs include sectorial microcystic corneal edema, irregular pupil, transillumination iris defect, low intraocular pressure, intraocular inflammation, or vitreous hemorrhages. Later findings include endophthalmitis, heterochromia, cataract, or corneal deposits.
- Substances such as vegetable, iron, copper, and steel may lead to intense inflammation or infection. Nickel, aluminum, and mercury tend to produce mild inflammation. Glass, carbon, porcelain, silver, and platinum are inert.

DIFFERENTIAL DIAGNOSIS

- Endophthalmitis and uveitis may mimic the findings of IOFB.

DIAGNOSTIC EVALUATION

- Orbital CT is the imaging modality of choice in detecting nonorganic IOFBs. Small organic foreign bodies such as wood or vegetable matter may escape detection.
- B-scan ultrasonography may detect IOFBs, retinal tears, or retinal detachments when the posterior pole cannot be visualized (Fig. 8-11B).
- Serial electroretinograms should be considered for retained metallic foreign bodies to evaluate for toxic metallosis.

PROGNOSIS AND MANAGEMENT

- Prognosis is largely dependent on the location and nature of the IOFB. Repair of the ruptured globe should be the first priority. Prompt removal of the IOFB via pars plana vitrectomy before 24 hours has been found to decrease the incidence of endophthalmitis.
- Considerations in the management of IOFBs include the following:
  - Always consider an IOFB masquerade syndrome in the setting of unilateral unexplained uveitis.
  - A CT scan with 1-mm sections through the globe and orbit is the best single imaging scan. MRI may be superior for imaging wood and organic material.

■ Copper, iron, and steel produce the most intense intraocular inflammatory response.

■ Surgical removal of intraocular foreign bodies is considered emergent and should be performed as soon as possible. Endophthalmitis associated with IOFBs is estimated up to 20%.

● Prompt surgical removal is recommended for vegetable, copper, iron, steel, or inert substances with toxic chemical coatings. Surgical extraction of certain metallic IOFBs may be facilitated by a magnet.

● Systemic and intravitreal antibiotics should be administered when there is a high index of suspicion for endophthalmitis.

FIGURE 8-11. Intraocular foreign body. A. Metallic foreign body in the retinal periphery. **B.** B-scan ultrasonography demonstrating acoustic shadowing (*arrow*) behind the intraocular foreign body.

DISLOCATED LENS

This term describes the total displacement of the native lens into the anterior chamber or the vitreous cavity as a result of lens zonular disruption.

EPIDEMIOLOGY

- The condition is most common in young males in the setting of trauma. Individuals with a familial or metabolic predisposition to zonular weakness are also prone to lens dislocation.

HISTORY

- There is usually a history of blunt ocular trauma. Often, the patient notes a dramatic decrease in visual acuity because of lens malposition.

CLINICAL SIGNS

- There is decreased vision, and the natural lens is seen in the anterior chamber or posterior pole (**Fig. 8-12**). Other signs associated with lens dislocation may include iridodonesis, irregular anterior chamber depth, eyelid ecchymosis, vitreous hemorrhage, or orbital fractures.

- The patient may have a physical habitus compatible with predisposing conditions such as Marfan's syndrome or Weill–Marchesani syndrome, among others.

DIFFERENTIAL DIAGNOSIS

- Conditions other than severe blunt trauma that predispose patients to lens dislocation include:

  - Marfan's syndrome: Patients are often tall and may have arachnodactyly.

Cardiac evaluation is important in evaluation for aortic aneurysm or insufficiency.

  - Weill–Marchesani syndrome: Affected individuals have short stature, seizures, microspherophakia, brachydactyly, and may have decreased hearing.

  - Homocystinuria: Patients may have marfanoid features, thrombosis (especially with general anesthesia), and below-average IQ.

  - Other: Syphilis, sulfite oxidase deficiency, high myopia, Ehlers–Danlos syndrome, and aniridia are other possible etiologies of lens dislocation.

DIAGNOSTIC EVALUATION

- B-scan ultrasonography is used in the setting of vitreous hemorrhage to evaluate for lens position and retinal detachment.

- Medical consultation is appropriate if Marfan's syndrome, homocystinuria, syphilis, or another predisposing condition is suspected.

PROGNOSIS AND MANAGEMENT

- Conservative management such as observation and contact lens wear may be considered. Management of dislocation of the natural lens into the anterior chamber causing glaucoma may include a trial of pupillary dilation and supine positioning in an attempt to dislocate the lens into the vitreous cavity.

- A lens that cannot be repositioned into the vitreous cavity or that has a disrupted lens capsule may require vitrectomy and lensectomy.

FIGURE 8-12. **Dislocated lens.** Intact native lens in the vitreous over a glaucomatous optic disc. (Courtesy of the Wills Eye Hospital collection, Philadelphia, Pennsylvania.)

TALC RETINOPATHY

Talc retinopathy describes the presence of an intraretinal, yellow, refractile substance in patients who abuse intravenous drugs, especially those using products made from crushed tablets or powder.

EPIDEMIOLOGY AND ETIOLOGY

• The condition can occur in persons of any age.

• The talc component of the injected medication migrates through microvascular venular to arteriolar shunts in the lungs and into the retinal arterioles.

HISTORY

• Patients have a history of chronic intravenous drug abuse. A history of intravenous injection of crushed methylphenidate (Ritalin) tablets may be elicited.

CLINICAL SIGNS

• Irregular refractile elements are seen throughout the retina (intravascular space), especially within the macula (**Fig. 8-13**).

• Other intraocular signs that may be seen include neovascularization of the retinal periphery (or optic nerve), macular pucker or fibrosis, or vitreous hemorrhage.

• Inspection of the skin may reveal evidence of intravenous drug abuse.

DIFFERENTIAL DIAGNOSIS

• The differential diagnosis for talc retinopathy includes other causes of crystalline retinopathy such as:

■ Canthaxanthin toxicity: Patients may volunteer a history of using oral tanning agents. The total cumulative dosage usually exceeds 19 g.

■ Tamoxifen (Nolvadex) use: Often there is a history of breast cancer and use of the antiestrogen agent for a cumulative dosage of at least 7.7 g.

• Retinal emboli associated with carotid obstructive disease or cardiac valve disease. Carotid ultrasonography or cardiac echography may reveal the embolic source.

• Intraretinal crystals

■ Talc particles (intravenous drug abuse)

■ Cholesterol (Hollenhorst plaque) or other emboli

■ Canthaxanthin ingestion (oral tanning agent)

■ Tamoxifen

■ Methoxyflurane anesthesia

■ Cystinosis

■ Parafoveal telangectasia (Singerman's dots)

■ Intraretinal lipid (hard exudates)

• Subretinal crystals (often associated with RPE alterations)

■ Calcified drusen

■ Bietti's corneal and macular crystalline dystrophy

DIAGNOSTIC EVALUATION

• Fluorescein angiography may reveal areas of nonperfusion in the retinal periphery.

• Optical coherence tomography may reveal hyperreflective bodies corresponding to inner retinal crystalline deposits.

PROGNOSIS AND MANAGEMENT

• The visual prognosis is variable. In the setting of chronic intravenous drug abuse, visual acuity may be decreased as a result of macular retinal capillary nonperfusion or vitreous hemorrhage.

• Decreased visual acuity may also occur secondary to macular fibrosis associated with intravenous methylphenidate abuse. Peripheral laser treatment can cause regression of retinal neovascularization.

FIGURE 8-13. **Talc retinopathy. A.** Color fundus photograph demonstrating yellow refractile particles within the retina. **B.** Red-free fundus photograph highlighting intraretinal macular refractile deposits.

CHLOROQUINE OR HYDROXYCHLOROQUINE RETINOPATHY

This entity describes degeneration of the RPE and neurosensory retinal damage resulting from chronic daily ingestion of chloroquine (Aralen) or hydroxychloroquine (Plaquenil).

EPIDEMIOLOGY

- The condition occurs in individuals receiving chloroquine for antimalarial treatment and in patients with rheumatoid arthritis or lupus erythematosus who take hydroxychloroquine. Hydroxychloroquine is less likely than chloroquine to cause retinopathy.

HISTORY

- There is a history of daily dosages exceeding 250 mg of chloroquine or 400 mg of hydroxychloroquine.

CLINICAL SIGNS

- Visual acuity is variable.
- An abnormal foveal reflex and subtle parafoveal retinal pigment epithelial stippling precedes the development of a ring of retinal pigment epithelial atrophy surrounding the foveal region, known as the classic "bull's-eye" maculopathy (Fig. 8-14). Retinal pigment epithelial disturbance underneath the fovea is associated with decreased visual acuity.
- A paracentral scotoma is the earliest sign of chloroquine or hydroxychloroquine toxicity and may precede the development of fundus findings.
- Other signs of chloroquine or hydroxychloroquine retinopathy include retinal vessel attenuation and corneal verticillata. Patients may display systemic findings of rheumatoid arthritis or lupus erythematosus.

DIFFERENTIAL DIAGNOSIS

- Cone dystrophy
- Chloroquine or hydroxychloroquine toxicity
- Benign concentric annular dystrophy
- Spielmeyer–Vogt–Batten disease
- Stargardt's maculopathy
- Age-related macular degeneration
- Fenestrated sheen macular dystrophy

DIAGNOSTIC EVALUATION

- Amsler grid evaluation may allow the patient to detect early scotoma formation.
- Humphrey visual field testing using red light may be the most sensitive means of detecting a paracentral scotoma.
- Color vision testing may reveal dyschromatopsia.
- Fluorescein angiography will show retinal pigment epithelial window defects in macular region.
- Electroretinography and electrooculography may be abnormal late findings.
- Optical coherence tomography may reveal thinning of macular and parafoveal retina with loss of ganglion cell layer.

PROGNOSIS AND MANAGEMENT

- Prompt discontinuation of medication on detection of toxicity usually prevents further damage to the RPE and retina.
- Patients with mild retinal pigment epithelial changes may revert to normal and retain good visual acuity. In advanced cases, however, the condition may worsen despite cessation of the medication, and visual loss may ensue.

FIGURE 8-14. Chloroquine retinopathy. A. Subtle parafoveal retinal pigment epithelial alterations (*arrow*) in a patient with a history of long-term chloroquine use. **B.** Bull's-eye maculopathy (inset) associated with chloroquine retinopathy. (**A,** Courtesy of Dr. Alexander J. Brucker; **B,** courtesy of the Wills Eye Hospital collection, Philadelphia, Pennsylvania.)

THIORIDAZINE RETINOPATHY

Thioridazine retinopathy describes visual disturbance and pigmentary retinopathy that results from chronic high-dose thioridazine use. Daily doses are more predictive of retinal toxicity than the total cumulative dose.

EPIDEMIOLOGY AND ETIOLOGY

• Individuals with psychiatric disorders requiring thioridazine.

• The exact mechanism of retinal damage is unclear although the medication is felt to accumulate in retinal pigment epithelial cells.

HISTORY

• The use of thioridazine (Mellaril) in excess of 800 mg per day has been associated with retinopathy.

CLINICAL SIGNS

• Acute toxicity is manifested by the sudden onset of visual disturbance, nyctalopia, or dyschromatopsia (red or brown coloration of vision). Retinal pigment epithelial changes can progress despite drug cessation.

• Early changes include granular retinal pigment epithelial stippling posterior to the equator.

• Nummular retinal pigment epithelial loss may be seen in intermediate stages (Fig. 8-15).

• Late features of thioridazine toxicity include optic atrophy, retinal vessel attenuation, diffuse RPE, and choriocapillaris atrophy.

DIFFERENTIAL DIAGNOSIS

• Gyrate atrophy, retinitis pigmentosa, cancer-associated retinopathy, choroideremia, syphilis, viral chorioretinitis, and trauma may demonstrate findings similar to thioridazine toxicity.

DIAGNOSTIC EVALUATION

• Humphrey visual field testing may reveal paracentral scotomas or constriction.

• Fluorescein angiography may reveal a spectrum of retinal pigment epithelial window defects and disruption of the choriocapillaris. The electroretinogram may be normal in early stages, but demonstrate attenuation in later stages.

PROGNOSIS AND MANAGEMENT

• Cessation of the drug early in the course of the toxicity may lead to reversal of visual disturbance. However, prolonged use of the medication may lead to progressive visual loss despite drug cessation.

FIGURE 8-15. Thioridazine retinopathy. A. Widespread retinal pigment epithelial and choriocapillaris atrophy. **B.** Less widespread retinal pigment epithelial and choriocapillaris atrophy may be mistaken for geographic atrophy due to age-related macular degeneration. Visual acuity is 20/200.

(continued)

FIGURE 8-15. (*Continued*) **Thioridazine retinopathy. C.** Fluorescein angiogram showing retinal pigment epithelial atrophy as well as nummular areas of choroidal vascular loss (*arrows*).

Peripheral Retinal Disease

James F. Vander

RETINAL BREAK OR TEAR

Retinal break or tear describes a full-thickness defect in the retina, generally in the retinal periphery, although the break may occur anywhere. Breaks occurring as the result of vitreous traction are known as retinal tears.

EPIDEMIOLOGY AND ETIOLOGY

- Retinal breaks are common. They are more frequent in myopia, pseudophakia, and after trauma.
- Many cases are bilateral and multiple.
- Retinal tears are caused by vitreous traction, most commonly found with degenerative vitreous liquefaction and posterior vitreous detachment (Fig. 9-1). Other retinal breaks (see later discussion) result from developmental or degenerative abnormalities or trauma.

HISTORY

- Retinal tears are often associated with floaters and flashing lights (photopsia).

- Many breaks are asymptomatic.
- If associated with retinal detachment (RD), then progressive visual field loss occurs.

IMPORTANT CLINICAL SIGNS

- Types of retinal breaks
  - Horseshoe (flap) tears: The horseshoe is open anteriorly. Vitreoretinal traction often persists (Fig. 9-2).
  - Operculated tears: A fragment of retina is torn completely free of the retina and floats above it. The vitreous traction is relieved (Fig. 9-3).
  - Atrophic retinal break: Usually round, often small, holes; not associated with traction (Fig. 9-4).
  - Retinal dialysis: Disinsertion of the retina from the pars plana at the ora serrata; most often inferotemporal; superonasal is virtually pathognomonic for trauma (Fig. 9-5).
  - Giant tear: A tear greater than 90 degrees, spontaneous or posttraumatic (Fig. 9-6).

■ Stretch/necrotic tears: Traumatic tears of variable size, often irregular in orientation with jagged edges; hemorrhage or other signs of trauma (Fig. 9-7).

ASSOCIATED CLINICAL SIGNS

• Look for predisposing conditions (see earlier discussion)

• Pigment cells in the vitreous ("tobacco dust")

• 70% with hemorrhagic posterior vitreous detachment (PVD)

• Vitreous hemorrhage [tears are found in 70% of patients with hemorrhagic proliferative vitreoretinopathy (PVR)]

• Subretinal fluid accumulating around the tear

• Pigment around the base of the retinal break (indicates chronicity)

DIFFERENTIAL DIAGNOSIS

• Vitreoretinal tuft
• Meridional fold or complex
• Outer wall hole in retinoschisis
• Cobblestone degeneration
• Lattice degeneration

DIAGNOSTIC EVALUATION

• Indirect ophthalmoscopy with scleral depression is critical.

• Contact lens examination of the periphery may help confirm the presence and nature of the break.

PROGNOSIS AND MANAGEMENT

• The risk of developing RD (and, therefore, indication for prophylactic treatment) depends on the type of break present. Symptomatic tears with persistent traction (horseshoe tears, giant tears) have a high risk of subsequent RD and are treated when recognized. Asymptomatic flap tears have a lower risk but are often prophylactically treated. Symptomatic operculated tears also have a much lower risk of subsequent RD.

• Treatment is more controversial. Dialysis and other posttraumatic tears are generally treated when recognized. Treatment for atrophic breaks, asymptomatic operculated tears, and breaks with pigment around them almost never require prophylactic treatment. Exceptions might include patients with a history of RD of the fellow eye, anticipated cataract surgery, or a strong family history of retinal tears or RD.

• Treatment options include cryotherapy or laser photocoagulation (Figs. 9-8–9-10). Development of the indirect ophthalmoscopic laser delivery system has facilitated the use of laser treatment and reduced the need for cryotherapy, which generally produces more pain during treatment. Patients with cloudy media or significant subretinal fluid may be better treated with cryotherapy.

FIGURE 9-1. Posterior vitreous detachment (PVD). A. Annulus of condensed vitreous (Weiss ring) (*arrow*) floating in front of the optic disc after PVD. **B.** Photograph focused on Weiss ring.

FIGURE 9-2. **Horseshoe retinal tear. A.** Horseshoe tear with a few flecks of hemorrhage and a small amount of subretinal fluid surrounding it. **B.** Large horseshoe tear with a bridging retinal vessel.

(*continued*)

FIGURE 9-2. (*Continued*) **Horseshoe retinal tear. C.** Horseshoe tear with associated retinal hemorrhages (*arrow*). Vitreous elevates the flap tear.

FIGURE 9-3. Operculated retinal tear.

FIGURE 9-4. **Peripheral cystoid degeneration.** Peripheral cystoid degeneration with associated atrophic retinal holes.

FIGURE 9-5. **Retinal dialysis.** Wide-angle view of inferotemporal dialysis with associated retinal detachment.

FIGURE 9-6. **Giant retinal tear.** Rolled edge of a giant retinal tear.

FIGURE 9-7. **Posttraumatic retinal tear. A.** Stretch tear after blunt trauma (*arrows* to retinal detachment).

(*continued*)

FIGURE 9-7. (*Continued*) **Posttraumatic retinal tear. B.** Two stretch tears after blunt trauma. **C.** Traumatic macular hole.

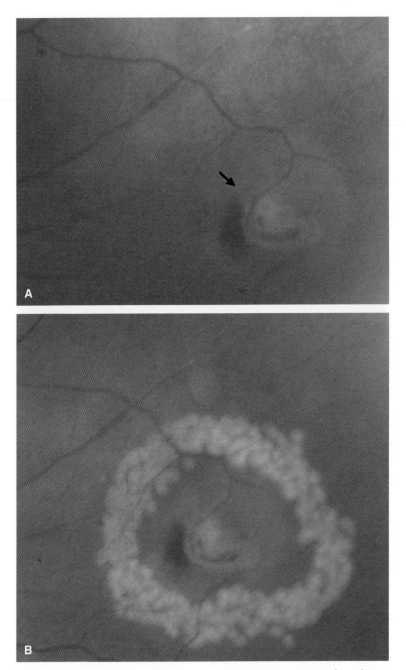

FIGURE 9-8. **Retinal tear, pretreatment and posttreatment. A.** Small horseshoe tear (*arrow*). **B.** Immediately after laser photocoagulation.

FIGURE 9-9. Retinal tear, pretreatment and posttreatment. A. Horseshoe tear with bridging vessel. **B.** Immediately after laser photocoagulation.

FIGURE 9-10. Retinal tear, posttreatment. A. Horseshoe retinal tear immediately after laser photocoagulation. **B.** Several weeks after laser photocoagulation for retinal tear in another patient. Laser marks have become pigmented.

RHEGMATOGENOUS RETINAL DETACHMENT

R hegmatogenous RD is a separation of the retina from the underlying retinal pigment epithelium (RPE) by fluid that gains access to the subretinal space via one or more full-thickness retinal breaks.

EPIDEMIOLOGY AND ETIOLOGY

• Epidemiology is the same as that for retinal breaks since, by definition, a retinal break is present and the cause of the RD.

• Retinal breaks develop into rhegmatogenous RD by a combination of vitreoretinal traction and fluid currents that cause vitreous fluid to move through the retinal break(s) and overcome the normal attractive forces between the photoreceptors and the RPE.

HISTORY

• There is a progressive loss of the visual field (often described as a curtain or shadow blocking the vision), frequently accompanied or preceded by floaters and flashing lights.

• Patients with peripheral RDs may be asymptomatic or simply have flashes and floaters.

IMPORTANT CLINICAL SIGNS

• In addition to identifying the retinal break(s), the retina is seen to be elevated by subretinal fluid (Fig. 9-11). The retina loses its transparency to a variable degree, often becoming translucent with a corrugated appearance. There is undulation with eye movement. Chronic rhegmatogenous RD may appear transparent and not undulate.

• Identifying the retinal break (often small and difficult to find) is the key. Pseudophakic RDs are often caused by small, pinpoint retinal holes at the vitreous base and may be difficult to detect.

ASSOCIATED CLINICAL SIGNS

• Pigment: Granules in the vitreous are almost always seen. Hyperpigmentation or loss of pigment at the RPE is common, especially in chronic RD. Linear pigment ("demarcation line") suggests chronicity and may be multiple (Fig. 9-12).

• Hypotony: Relative to the fellow eye. This is not invariably present. In chronic rhegmatogenous RD, pressure may be normal or even high.

• Other features of chronic RD: Retinal neovascularization, cataract, anterior uveitis, rubeosis iridis, and retinal cysts (Fig. 9-13).

DIFFERENTIAL DIAGNOSIS

• Retinoschisis
• Exudative RD
• Tractional RD
• Choroidal detachment

DIAGNOSTIC EVALUATION

• Indirect ophthalmoscopy with scleral depression is the key. Contact lens examination may help find small peripheral retinal breaks.

• Slit-lamp examination of the anterior vitreous confirms vitreous pigment.

• B-scan ultrasonography confirms retinal elevation in cases with media opacities.

• Examine the fellow eye to look for retinoschisis.

PROGNOSIS

- Chronic, asymptomatic RD may remain stationary and not require treatment.

- Spontaneous regression of RD can occur but is rare (Fig. 9-14).

- Most RDs and virtually all symptomatic detachments will progress, causing severe permanent visual loss if untreated. Visual potential is directly related to the presence and duration of macular involvement (Fig. 9-15).

- RDs not involving the macula often recover vision fully.

- "Macula-off" RDs usually lead to permanent reduction of central vision even when repaired properly. Recovery often takes months, and the degree of recovery diminishes with longer periods of macular detachment.

Management

- Laser photocoagulation: Used alone it has a limited role in management of RD. Usually it cannot seal a retinal break closed in the presence of subretinal fluid. Laser treatment may be used to create a barrier ("wall off the detachment") to prevent progression of the detachment. It is especially useful in chronic inferior RD or in cases where systemic illness prevents more definitive repair.

- Cryotherapy (see preceding discussion of Laser Photocoagulation): Occasionally RDs with very shallow fluid around the retinal break can be cured by treating the break with cryotherapy alone.

- Pneumatic retinopexy: An intravitreal gas bubble is used to tamponade the retinal break closed temporarily. The subretinal fluid will resolve and either laser photocoagulation or cryotherapy is used to permanently close the retinal break(s). The success rate is high and varies with patient selection. Patients with phakic RDs with a single, superior retinal break without vitreous hemorrhage, extensive lattice degeneration, or early PVR do best. This relatively noninvasive, low-cost, quick-recovery office procedure is gaining in acceptance.

- Temporary balloon: This treatment consists of an external device applied via small conjunctival incisions. The balloon temporarily indents the sclera to allow cryotherapy or a laser-induced chorioretinal adhesion to form. This treatment option is especially useful for inferior RD when pneumatic retinopexy is not an option; however, it is not a widely used technique.

- Scleral buckle: This widely applied technique consists of indentation of the sclera using a flexible silicone sponge or strip that is permanently sutured on or within the sclera to relieve vitreoretinal traction on the retinal break(s). Cryotherapy is generally used to create permanent adhesion although postoperative laser therapy can be applied. Drainage of subretinal fluid or injection of intravitreal gas, or both, are also sometimes performed to assist in reattachment. Success rates of over 95% have been reported for repair of primary RD. Side effects and complications of the scleral buckle include:

  - Pain
  - Infection
  - Hemorrhage (especially with drainage of subretinal fluid; Fig. 9-16)
  - Retinal incarceration at drainage site (Fig. 9-17)
  - Induced myopia
  - Diplopia
  - Extrusion or intrusion (Fig. 9-18)
  - Anterior segment ischemia
  - Ptosis

- Vitrectomy: This technique is increasingly used in managing primary RD with or without a scleral buckle. It allows for direct release of vitreoretinal traction. Intravitreal gas or silicone oil is used to tamponade the retina while retinopexy with laser or cryotherapy takes effect. Vitrectomy is especially useful for RDs with posterior breaks, PVR, vitreous hemorrhage, or a tight orbit preventing scleral buckle. Side effects and complications of vitrectomy include:

- Elevated intraocular pressure
- Cataract
- Dislocation of intraocular lens
- Infection
- Hemorrhage
- Postoperative positioning (e.g., face-down) may be needed

FIGURE 9-11. **Rhegmatogenous retinal detachment (RD). A.** Rhegmatogenous RD with a small horseshoe tear (*arrow*).

(*continued*)

FIGURE 9-11. (*Continued*) **Rhegmatogenous retinal detachment (RD). B.** RD with bullous elevation and corrugated appearance of the detached retina. **C.** RD with a small horseshoe tear (*arrow*).

FIGURE 9-12. Rhegmatogenous RD, chronic. A. Chronic RD (*right of arrows*) with pigmented demarcation line (*arrows*). **B.** Chronic RD (*black arrow*) with multiple demarcation lines and some subretinal fibrous bands (*white arrows*).

FIGURE 9-13. Rhegmatogenous RD, chronic. A. Retinal cysts associated with chronic RD. **B.** B-scan ultrasound of retinal cyst (*short arrow*) and chronic RD (*long arrow*).

FIGURE 9-14. **Rhegmatogenous RD, regressed.** Pigmentation from spontaneously regressed RD.

FIGURE 9-15. **Rhegmatogenous RD, pigmentary disturbances.** Subretinal dispersion of pigment after repair of "macula-off" RD.

FIGURE 9-16. Rhegmatogenous RD, subretinal hemorrhage. A. Subretinal hemorrhage beneath the attached retina associated with drainage of subretinal fluid during scleral buckling surgery. **B.** Macular extension of subretinal blood complicating drainage of subretinal fluid.

FIGURE 9-17. **Rhegmatogenous RD, retinal incarceration.** Incarceration of the retina into the drainage site during scleral buckle.

FIGURE 9-18. **Scleral buckle.** Extruding scleral buckle.

PROLIFERATIVE VITREORETINOPATHY

● PVR refers to the development of preretinal, subretinal, and even intraretinal fibrous proliferation that induces traction and distortion of the retina in the presence of RD (**Table 9-1**).

EPIDEMIOLOGY AND ETIOLOGY

● In the presence of RD, activation of vitreous glial cells and metaplasia of retinal pigment epithelial cells produces fibrous tissue that proliferates on and under the retina.

● Although the mechanism is not totally understood, risk factors include RDs with multiple retinal breaks, large retinal breaks, chronicity, vitreous hemorrhage, and trauma.

TABLE 9-1. Classification of Proliferative Vitreoretinopathy

Grade A	Vitreous haze, vitreous pigment clumps, and pigment clusters inferior to retina
Grade B	Inner retinal wrinkling, retinal stiffness, vessel tortuosity, rolled edge of break, and decreased vitreous mobility
Grade C	P (posterior)—expressed in the number of clock hours involved (1–12)
	Focal, diffuse, or circumferential full-thickness folds, subretinal strands
	A (anterior)—expressed in the number of clock hours involved (1–12)
	Focal, diffuse, or circumferential full-thickness folds; subretinal strands; condensed vitreous; and anterior displacement of vitreous base with anterior trough.

● PVR may be primary or develop after attempted repair of RD. It tends to occur 3 weeks to 3 months after initial repair.

HISTORY

● The same as for RD.

IMPORTANT CLINICAL SIGNS

● The retina is relatively immobile with fixed folds.

● Rolled edges of the retinal break(s) and extensive pigment in vitreous, on and under retina are noted (**Fig. 9-19**).

● Vitreous bands are prominent.

ASSOCIATED CLINICAL SIGNS

● Hypotony
● Anterior flare or uveitis
● Rubeosis iridis

DIFFERENTIAL DIAGNOSIS

● Purely tractional RD (e.g., diabetic retinopathy; **Fig. 9-20**)
● Exudative RD

DIAGNOSTIC EVALUATION

● Diagnosis is based on indirect ophthalmoscopy.

● Ultrasound may show the rigid nature of RD if detachment cannot be directly visualized.

PROGNOSIS AND MANAGEMENT

- PVR almost always progresses, causing severe visual loss. Repair is difficult, especially for more advanced degrees of PVR (see **Table 9-1**).

- Repair almost always includes vitrectomy, often with a high encircling scleral buckle as well as a long-lasting vitreous gas or silicone oil tamponade.

- Recurrence rate is high, and recovery of excellent visual acuity is uncommon in severe cases (**Figs. 9-21 and 9-22**).

FIGURE 9-19. Proliferative vitreoretinopathy (PVR). A. High magnification view of PVR with radiating retinal folds. **B.** Wide field view showing retinal folds radiating from optic disc.

FIGURE 9-20. **Tractional RD associated with proliferative diabetic retinopathy.** Wide-field view of traction retinal detachment with regressed neovascularization producing a ring of fibrotic traction.

FIGURE 9-21. **PVR, recurrent RD.** Recurrent RD with severe PVR. Note severe fibrous proliferation on the retinal surface and associated retinal breaks.

FIGURE 9-22. PVR, fixed retinal folds. A. PVR with macular pucker (*long arrow*) after vitrectomy and scleral buckle for RD. Note the edge of the slowly clearing vitreous gas bubble (*short arrow*) used during the initial repair. **B.** Inferior proliferation causing tractional elevation of the retina (*arrow*).

LATTICE DEGENERATION

Lattice degeneration is a peripheral fundus abnormality consisting of retinal thinning with loss of inner retinal tissue and unusually strong vitreoretinal adhesion at the edges of the retinal excavation.

EPIDEMIOLOGY AND ETIOLOGY

● The condition is common, occurring in about 8% of the population. It is more common and more extensive in patients with myopia.

HISTORY

● Patients are asymptomatic except when the condition is associated with retinal tear and detachment formation.

IMPORTANT CLINICAL SIGNS

● Lattice degeneration can be variable in pigmentation, circumferential extent, and orientation (usually concentric with ora serrata but may be radial or perivascular) (Fig. 9-23).
● Cross-hatched white lines, which give the appearance of a lattice, are often not present. Indirect ophthalmoscopy is usually necessary to see lattice degeneration.
● Dynamic scleral depression is the key to appreciating the inner retinal excavation.

ASSOCIATED CLINICAL SIGNS

● Myopia
● Stickler's syndrome: This syndrome, which has an autosomal-dominant

inheritance, consists of vitreoretinopathy with arthropathy and other systemic features.
● Retinal breaks: Atrophic round holes are often present within the lattice degeneration, sometimes with associated subretinal fluid. Tractional flap tears may occur, usually at the edges of the lattice (Fig. 9-24).

DIFFERENTIAL DIAGNOSIS

● Cobblestone degeneration
● Cystoid degeneration
● Retinoschisis
● Vitreoretinal tuft
● Pigmented or atrophic chorioretinal scars
● Grouped pigmentation

DIAGNOSTIC EVALUATION

● Indirect ophthalmoscopy is performed with scleral depression.
● Peripheral contact lens examination may help confirm the presence of associated tears.

PROGNOSIS AND MANAGEMENT

● Usually this condition is of no clinical significance.
● The risk of RD increases with the extent of lattice degeneration. Prophylactic treatment (laser or cryotherapy) generally is not indicated except if the fellow eye had lattice-related RD.
● A strong family history of retinal tear or RD or anticipated intraocular surgery are other possible considerations for treatment.

FIGURE 9-23. **Pigmented lattice degeneration.** Note the lattice-like network within the area of increased pigmentation.

FIGURE 9-24. **Lattice degeneration with associated horseshoe tear and RD (*arrow*).** A horseshoe tear at the edge of lattice reflects firm vitreoretinal adhesion at the edge of the lattice degeneration.

VITREORETINAL TUFT AND MERIDIONAL FOLD

Vitreoretinal tuft and meridional fold are common structural abnormalities of the extreme retinal periphery with unusually strong vitreoretinal adhesion. They are infrequently the cause of rhegmatogenous RD.

EPIDEMIOLOGY AND ETIOLOGY

- Vitreoretinal tufts are very common in the general population and are the source of RD in less than 1% of all affected patients.
- Meridional folds are very common in the general population and are the source of RD in less than 1% of all affected patients.
- They are a developmental abnormality.

HISTORY

- The abnormalities are asymptomatic except when they precipitate RD.

IMPORTANT CLINICAL SIGNS

- Vitreoretinal tufts are small areas of substantial focal vitreous traction producing a discrete retinal elevation (Fig. 9-25). There may be pigment around the tuft. They often are mistaken for small flap tears, but no full-thickness break is present.
- Meridional folds are folds of redundant retina (Fig. 9-26). Most often superonasal, they may straddle and are perpendicular to the ora serrata. Small retinal breaks may develop at their posterior end.

DIFFERENTIAL DIAGNOSIS

- Retinal tear
- "Snowball" or other inflammatory precipitate

PROGNOSIS AND MANAGEMENT

- Both abnormalities are almost always incidental findings of no clinical importance.
- Rarely, they may be the only abnormal finding in cases of RD and are presumed to be the cause of the detachment.
- They are generally treated with cryotherapy or laser photocoagulation at the time of RD repair, but prophylactic treatment is not warranted.

FIGURE 9-25. **Vitreoretinal tuft.** Focal opacification and elevation of the retina occurs at two gray-white vitreoretinal tufts.

FIGURE 9-26. **Schematic of meridional fold.** The fold represents a pleat of retina between the ora bays.

COBBLESTONE DEGENERATION

Cobblestone degeneration, also called paving stone degeneration, describes discrete circular areas of peripheral atrophy of the retina, RPE, and choriocapillaris.

EPIDEMIOLOGY AND ETIOLOGY

- This is a degenerative process of unknown etiology.
- The condition is more common in the elderly.

HISTORY

- Patients are usually asymptomatic.

IMPORTANT CLINICAL SIGNS

- Circular areas of thinning of the retina with depigmentation are seen (Fig. 9-27).

- Often a pigmented halo is noted.
- The degeneration is most common inferiorly and is usually bilateral.

DIFFERENTIAL DIAGNOSIS

- Retinal breaks
- Lattice degeneration
- Congenital hypertrophy of RPE

DIAGNOSTIC EVALUATION

- Diagnosis is based on indirect ophthalmoscopy.

PROGNOSIS AND MANAGEMENT

- Cobblestone degeneration is of no clinical importance. It is not a predisposing condition for RD and, in fact, may be protective against a progressive RD.

FIGURE 9-27. **Cobblestone (paving stone) degeneration.** Areas of pigmentation are observed within the discrete areas of depigmentation.

PERIPHERAL GROUPED PIGMENTATION

Peripheral grouped pigmentation describes a cluster of flat, discrete pigmented spots deep to retina.

EPIDEMIOLOGY AND ETIOLOGY

- It may occur at any age, in both genders.
- This is a congenital abnormality.

HISTORY

- Patients are usually asymptomatic.

IMPORTANT CLINICAL SIGNS

- A cluster of flat, uniformly pigmented spots of variable size are often noted (Fig. 9-28). These are also known as "bear tracks" because of their paw-print appearance. Rarely, the pigmentation is bilateral.

ASSOCIATED CLINICAL SIGNS

- There are no signs of inflammation, fluid, or elevation.

DIFFERENTIAL DIAGNOSIS

- Cobblestone degeneration
- Choroidal nevus or melanoma
- Lattice degeneration
- Chorioretinal scar
- Important: Peripheral grouped pigmentation must be distinguished from the pigmented spots in the fundus that are seen in familial polyposis (Gardner's syndrome). This autosomal-dominant condition, which is usually asymptomatic, often includes flat, variably pigmented spots in the fundus. Lesions of Gardner's syndrome tend to be more oval, with an irregularly pigmented "comet's tail" (Fig. 9-29). Affected patients have a very high risk of colonic carcinoma. Fundus lesions in Gardner's syndrome are usually seen as early as infancy. For patients with a positive family history, the presence of fundus lesions is virtually diagnostic of the systemic syndrome.

DIAGNOSTIC EVALUATION

- Diagnosis is based on indirect ophthalmoscopy.
- For suspicious lesions (see preceding discussion), obtain a family history of gastrointestinal malignancy and consider colonoscopy.

PROGNOSIS AND MANAGEMENT

- Peripheral grouped pigmentation is of no clinical importance with no potential for RD or malignant transformation.

FIGURE 9-28. **Grouped pigmentation.** Small clumps of grouped pigmentation ("bear tracks"; inset) have little risk of malignant transformation.

FIGURE 9-29. **Pigmented fundus lesions associated with Gardner's syndrome.** Note the depigmented halo (*arrowhead*) and oblong shape of the lesion.

DEGENERATIVE RETINOSCHISIS

- Degenerative retinoschisis is a splitting of the retina that produces elevation of the inner retina, mimicking a detachment.

EPIDEMIOLOGY AND ETIOLOGY

- The condition is a degenerative process that begins with peripheral cystoid degeneration. Further splitting in the outer plexiform layer leads to the elevation noted clinically.
- Degenerative retinoschisis affects both genders and all races.

HISTORY

- Patients are asymptomatic except in rare cases of progressive RD.

IMPORTANT CLINICAL SIGNS

- A transparent dome-shaped elevation of peripheral retina may be easily overlooked (Fig. 9-30).
- A thin, cystic appearance is noted.
- The inferotemporal fundus is most often affected. In the majority of cases the condition is bilateral.
- The retina is immobile, and there is no associated pigmentation of the RPE or vitreous.

ASSOCIATED CLINICAL SIGNS

- White "snowflakes" on the underside of the inner retinal layer or a pockmarked appearance may be noted.
- Outer wall holes are circular, and there are sometimes multiple defects (Fig. 9-31).

- Detection of an intact, overlying, inner layer is facilitated by noting retinal vessels coursing over the hole.
- An absolute visual field defect corresponds to the area of retinoschisis.

DIFFERENTIAL DIAGNOSIS

- Rhegmatogenous RD: The presence of a retinal break, corrugations, undulations, pigment in vitreous or demarcation lines, symptoms, hypotony, and a fellow eye that is normal help distinguish this condition from retinoschisis.
- Exudative RD: Associated tumor or inflammatory signs, shifting fluid, and symptoms suggest this etiology.
- Juvenile retinoschisis (X-linked): This heritable condition produces a stellate foveal appearance with splitting neurosensory retina within the nerve fiber layer. It may present as vitreous hemorrhage.

DIAGNOSTIC EVALUATION

- Evaluation consists of indirect ophthalmoscopy with scleral depression and contact lens examination.
- The fellow eye should also be examined.

PROGNOSIS AND MANAGEMENT

- Degenerative retinoschisis rarely produces vision loss. Progression to posterior retina or development of true rhegmatogenous detachment is uncommon.
- Outer wall defects usually are easily detected, but inner wall breaks are difficult to identify. In cases of very posterior retinoschisis with progression, outer wall breaks may be surrounded with laser treatment (Fig. 9-32).
- If the outer layer is detached as well, then surgery, usually vitrectomy, is needed.

FIGURE 9-30. Peripheral retinoschisis. A. Note the smooth, dome-shaped elevation in the inferotemporal quadrant (*arrows*). **Degenerative retinoschisis B.** Wide-angle photograph of inferotemporal retinoschisis (lower left). The external transillumination is noted (directly left).

FIGURE 9-31. Degenerative retinoschisis, outer wall breaks. Outer wall holes associated with retinoschisis (inset) are required to cause a retinoschisis-associated retinal detachment. Note that the inner-layer retinal vessels course over the outer-layer retinal holes.

FIGURE 9-32. Degenerative retinoschisis, outer wall breaks. Laser treatment (*arrows*) surrounding outer wall holes (asterisks) in retinoschisis.

EXUDATIVE RETINAL DETACHMENT

Exudative RD describes elevation of the retina by fluid that leaks from within or under the retina.

EPIDEMIOLOGY AND ETIOLOGY

- By definition, the retinal elevation is not due to a retinal break.
- Breakdown of the normal inner (retinal vascular endothelial cells) or outer blood–retinal barrier (RPE) produces exudation of fluid, elevating the retina.
- Cases can be divided into one of four categories, as follows:
  - **Inflammatory**
    - ▸ Scleritis
    - ▸ Harada's disease
    - ▸ Sympathetic ophthalmia
    - ▸ Orbital pseudotumor and other orbital inflammation
    - ▸ Infectious retinochoroiditis (e.g., toxoplasmosis, syphilis, Lyme disease, bartonellosis)
    - ▸ Vasculitis or autoimmune (e.g., lupus, polyarteritis nodosa)
  - **Vascular**
    - ▸ Coats' disease (Fig. 9-33)
    - ▸ Retinal capillary hemangioma
    - ▸ Acute systemic hypertension
    - ▸ Eclampsia
    - ▸ Disseminated intravascular coagulation (DIC)
    - ▸ Renal failure
  - **Neoplastic**
    - ▸ Choroidal melanoma (Fig. 9-34)
    - ▸ Choroidal metastasis
    - ▸ Retinoblastoma
  - **Miscellaneous**
    - ▸ Bullous central serous choroidopathy
    - ▸ Uveal effusion syndrome
    - ▸ Nanophthalmos
    - ▸ Coloboma

HISTORY

- Patients experience a progressive, often fluctuating loss of peripheral vision, that is similar to rhegmatogenous RD, but often more variable in course.
- Visual changes may be positional, caused by shifting subretinal fluid with changes in head position.
- If inflammatory in nature, the condition may cause pain; however, it is often asymptomatic.

IMPORTANT CLINICAL SIGNS

- There is a dome-shaped elevation of the retina, which retains its transparency (Fig. 9-35).
- The subretinal fluid generally shifts to the most gravity-dependent position with changes in the patient's head position.

ASSOCIATED CLINICAL SIGNS

- Observe for features of the underlying cause, such as inflammation, vascular changes, or solid tumor (see Fig. 9-34).

DIFFERENTIAL DIAGNOSIS

- Rhegmatogenous RD (especially chronic with small retinal break) differential diagnosis

- Retinoschisis
- Choroidal detachment

DIAGNOSTIC EVALUATION

- Fluorescein angiography: Often shows source(s) of subretinal fluid and the nature of the defect causing it (see discussion under "Epidemiology and Etiology," earlier).
- B-scan ultrasound: Thickening of sclera is seen in scleritis or orbital inflammation.

Calcification suggests retinoblastoma. Identify features of choroidal tumor or thickening.

- A-scan ultrasound: Short axial length is typical of nanophthalmos.

PROGNOSIS AND MANAGEMENT

- The prognosis varies markedly, depending on the underlying etiology. Treatment depends on the underlying cause.

FIGURE 9-33. **Exudative RD associated with Coats' disease (*arrow*).** Note the subretinal lipid precipitates where the exudative RD is shallower.

FIGURE 9-34. **Exudative RD overlying choroidal melanoma with retinal hemorrhages.** This smooth, dome-shaped elevation extends beyond the choroidal melanoma.

CHOROIDAL DETACHMENT

Choroidal detachment refers to elevation of the retina and choroid by either accumulation of serous fluid or blood in the suprachoroidal space.

EPIDEMIOLOGY AND ETIOLOGY

- Serous choroidal detachment is generally a secondary effect of another underlying problem.
- Causes include:
  - Hypotony
  - Wound leak
  - Postglaucoma surgery
  - Cyclodialysis cleft
  - Inflammation
  - High scleral buckle
- Hemorrhagic choroidal detachment may occur spontaneously, intraoperatively after trauma, or as the result of vascular abnormalities such as choroidal neovascularization.

HISTORY

- Occurrence of a visual field defect or shadow may be gradual or sudden in onset.
- There may be associated severe pain, if hemorrhagic.

IMPORTANT CLINICAL SIGNS

- A dome-shaped elevation of the retina and choroid is noted. The retina and choroid may appear normal in every way except for their relative position within the eye.
- If large enough, the detachment may obstruct the examiner's view of the optic nerve and macula. If elevations are very large, they may contact each other in vitreous cavity ("kissing choroidals").

ASSOCIATED CLINICAL SIGNS

- Hypotony
- Marked elevation of intraocular pressure (hemorrhagic choroidals)
- Vitreous hemorrhage
- Retinal folds or detachment
- Shallow anterior chamber

DIFFERENTIAL DIAGNOSIS

- Choroidal melanoma
- Choroidal metastasis
- RD
- Retinoschisis
- Scleral buckle

DIAGNOSTIC EVALUATION

- If choroidal detachment is associated with hypotony, look for the cause (e.g., gonioscopy for cyclodialysis cleft).
- B-scan ultrasonography confirms the diagnosis and helps distinguish between serous and hemorrhagic detachment. It also will show evidence of inflammation of the sclera or orbit, and can help distinguish detachment from neoplasm.

PROGNOSIS AND MANAGEMENT

- The prognosis for patients with serous choroidal detachment is generally favorable if the underlying etiology can be reversed.

Restoration of normal intraocular pressure and eradication of inflammation are generally adequate to reverse this process.

- Hemorrhagic detachment can produce severe pain or marked elevation of intraocular pressure requiring prompt surgical drainage. Otherwise, the condition can generally be observed and will slowly resolve.

- If the vitreous or retina is adherent to anterior structures such as a cataract wound, vitrectomy is indicated or else RD will occur as the choroidal detachment resolves.

- Surgical drainage is usually recommended for "kissing choroidals," although the necessity and optimal timing of this procedure are controversial.

FIGURE 9-35. **Exudative RD.** This detachment exhibited shifting subretinal fluid with change of position.

Index

Note: Page numbers followed by *f* and *t* indicate figures and tables, respectively.